Inconceivable

INCONCEIVABLE

My Life-Altering, Eye-Opening Journey from Infertility to Motherhood

ALEX JOHNSTON

sh.

SUTHERLAND HOUSE

TORONTO, 2021

Sutherland House
416 Moore Ave., Suite 205
Toronto, ON M4G 1C9

First edition, May 2021

If you are interested in inviting one of our authors to a live event or media appearance, please contact publicity@sutherlandhousebooks.com and visit our website at sutherlandhousebooks.com for more information about our authors and their schedules.

Manufactured in Canada
Cover designed by Lena Yang
Book composed by Karl Hunt
Library and Archives Canada Cataloguing in Publication
Title: Inconceivable : My Life-Altering, Eye-Opening Journey from Infertility to Motherhood / Alex Johnston.
Names: Johnston, Alex, 1970- author.
Identifiers: Canadiana 20200377027 |
ISBN 9781989555392 (softcover)
Subjects: LCSH: Johnston, Alex, 1970- | LCSH: Johnston, Alex, 1970—Health. | LCSH: Infertility, Female. | LCSH: Infertility, Female—Social aspects. | LCSH: Infertility, Female—Psychological aspects. | LCSH: Fertilization in vitro, Human. | LCSH: Surrogate motherhood. | LCSH: Reproductive health services. | LCGFT: Autobiographies.
Classification: LCC RG201 .J64 2021 | DDC 362.1981/780092—dc23

ISBN 978-1-989555-39-2

TABLE OF CONTENTS

This book is dedicated to Debbie and Diane.

With thanks and love.

The Canadian author royalties from this book will be donated to two organizations that have worked so hard for so many years to better our awareness and understanding of infertility. Fertility Matters and Conceivable Dreams are tireless advocates for the necessary policy and funding changes to support women and men who need help building their families. I don't know what will come from sharing my story, but I hope it will help to amplify their exceptional work.

Visit them at FertilityMatters.ca and ConceivableDreams.org

PREFACE

THERE'S A MOVIE FROM THE 1990S, *Sliding Doors*, where Gwyneth Paltrow stars as a woman who lives two different hypothetical lives. There's a critical juncture in the movie where she runs to get on a subway car just as the doors are closing. The first half of the movie shows you what unfolds in the version where she gets on. The second half shows you an alternate version where she doesn't. The subway doors close and she returns home to find her partner in bed with another woman, setting her life on a very different path.

Over the many years I spent struggling to have children, I experienced many sliding-doors moments. I often wanted to rewind the clock and, with the benefit of knowledge, go back and steer to a different destination.

Of course, you can't turn back the clock. But you can pay your experiences forward, which is what I hope to do with my infertility experience and why I am sharing my story.

Mine is by no means a typical journey, if there is such a thing. I discovered quickly, for instance, that infertility treatment is expensive. I was lucky enough to have been able to afford help—lots of it. I know how privileged I was to have been in a position to pursue different options to try to build my family. That's another reason I'm writing this book: to share the benefits of my expensive infertility education so that others can make their journeys more affordable.

Otherwise, parts of my story are likely to be very relatable for many women who have gone through infertility treatment. Infertility robbed me of my thirties. It extracted a toll on my career, my marriage, my family relationships, and my friendships. I hear people talk about how great their thirties were—building their families and careers. For me, a lot of that decade is a blur.

Infertility is an even bigger issue today than when I was going through it. When I started trying to get pregnant in 2003, the average age of childbirth in Canada, where I live, was twenty-nine.[1] Now it is thirty-one. Of the almost 400,000 babies born in Canada in 2019,[2] the majority of these were born to mothers in their thirties, which has been the case since 2010.[3] Since 2016, the majority of babies in the U.S. have been born to women in their thirties.[4]

The age of pregnancy is highly influenced by education. In the U.S., the median age of a first birth is thirty for women with master's degrees, twenty-eight for those with bachelor's degrees, twenty-five for those who have attended a college, and twenty-four for those with a high school education or less.[5]

Connected to these demographic shifts, infertility treatment has become a booming business over the past twenty years. In 2001, twenty fertility clinics in Canada initiated 7,844 In Vitro Fertilization (IVF) cycles.[6] By 2017, that number had grown to thirty-six clinics and 33,092 cycles.[7] The use of assisted reproductive technology in the U.S. has almost doubled over the past decade.[8] IVF is a $20 billion (US) dollar a year global industry today, and projected to grow to almost $38 billion by 2027.[9]

These same pregnancy trends are taking place everywhere. In Japan, Ireland, Italy, Korea, Luxembourg, Spain and Switzerland, the average age of childbirth is now over thirty-two.[10] These shifts are significant because by the age of thirty-two a woman's fertility has started a gradual but significant decline.[11]

Infertility is a more public topic now than it was when I was going through it. Many celebrities have shared their struggles publicly. It has been written into storylines on popular sitcoms. Influential public figures like Michelle Obama have been open about using fertility treatments to have their children. Magazines regularly profile celebrities who are having children well into their forties. But they don't explain that getting pregnant at that age with your own eggs, even with fertility help, is like getting hit by lightning. It happens, but very rarely.

An unfortunate side-effect of infertility discussions entering the mainstream is that too many people are getting their information from popular culture. This can create harmful misperceptions, making it look easier to get pregnant or to get help than it actually is. There are indeed more options today for fertility preservation, such as egg freezing. These are being aggressively marketed to younger women as a panacea, but the reality is that few women have the money or the health insurance coverage to afford these options.

All of this leaves women with the erroneous impression that pregnancy can happen at any age, which simply isn't true.

I have focused this book on women. When I talk about infertility, people often say, "But men's fertility declines too." That is true. But men's fertility starts to decline much later, in their forties, well past the age when most men are having children. It is also much easier to identify and address infertility in men, through much less invasive and expensive means, than it is to treat infertility in women.

That is not to say that this issue isn't equally important for men. Men and women together are choosing to have children later. They will confront the reality of a woman's biological clock together. Men, as much as women, need to be fully engaged in this discussion.

So while a deeper and more public conversation about infertility is beginning, we still aren't confronting the prevalence or significance of the problem with any sense of urgency. That needs to change.

Sharing my story is not meant to scare women or pressure them into having babies before they are ready. Becoming a parent is a deeply personal choice. Women should be able to make a choice that is right for them. Choice is sacred.

But to be able to make that choice, I want women to be armed with the right information so that they don't wake up one day and realize that a door has already quietly closed before they even had a chance to consider opening it.

I don't want my path for other women. If nothing else comes from telling my story, I want young women who may want a child one day to be able to preserve their choice.

For that to happen, we need to get over whatever discomfort we have in addressing infertility—whether it is shame, blame, pain, guilt, ignorance, embarrassment, fear, or just plain inertia—and face the issues frankly and honestly.

This is my story.

Housekeeping Items . . .

You will meet my parents and my four sisters in this book so I am introducing them at the outset to help keep them straight.

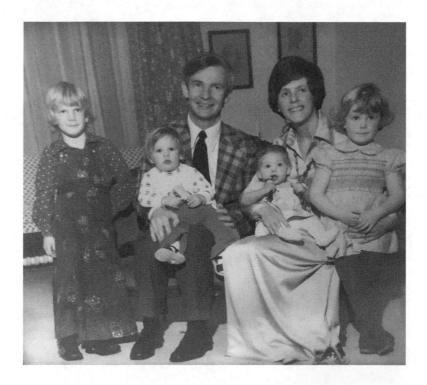

This is my favourite childhood photo. We seem to have dressed to match our living room furniture. Mom and Dad, Deb (left, wearing a jean dress that she made herself), Sharon (Dad's lap), Jen (mom's lap) and me (right). My mom was pregnant with Sam, who will be mad that I chose a photo without her, so I have added her here.

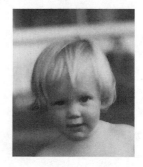

You will also meet my husband David.

We met in university while taking a women's history class where he was one of two men in a class of hundreds. Even with those odds, I didn't notice him until he "randomly" started to study at the same campus library where I studied and "coincidentally" took his breaks when I took mine. He describes our courtship as a long one involving a lot of tea and talking, and not much else. That's a fair characterization. When I finally let him start sleeping over at my apartment, months into dating, I wore a track suit to bed each night. I didn't want him to get the wrong idea.

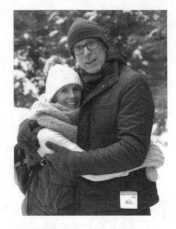

But he persevered and I am the luckier for it.

CHAPTER ONE

Do As I Say,
Not As I Do

W HEN I WAS THIRTY-TWO YEARS OLD, David and I sat on a balcony in Italy talking about our future. We made a decision to start building our family.

We had been married for eight months. I didn't feel ready to let go of our life without kids, but I also knew that I had a biological clock and I didn't want to end up as one of those women who waited too long and had trouble getting pregnant.

I made an appointment with my family doctor when I got home from our trip. She gave me the standard advice for women my age: try for twelve months. It never crossed my mind that I would have any trouble. My mom had five girls in seven years. With all that estrogen in our house growing up, fertility didn't seem to be an issue.

I spent the first few months joking with friends about how much sex I was going to have. I spent the next few months wondering if David was doing it wrong. Eighteen months after the balcony conversation, I was standing in a fertility clinic listening to my fertility specialist tell me that things didn't look good. My fertility work-up had just come back: my hormone levels were borderline menopausal and my ovaries didn't have many eggs left.

I was shocked and asked how that was possible. I was only thirty-four. She explained that twenty percent of women my age were infertile. I was speechless. I probably should have known that I was in for a rough ride when I did an ultrasound for my fertility work-up; I asked the technician what the dark empty circles were on the screen and she said, "Those are your ovaries".

How had I not known any of this important information?

I had a good family doctor but I don't think we ever discussed fertility until I told her that I was ready to start a family. As I learned the facts about infertility, it baffled me that every girl and woman would not be equipped early in life with information on how to reduce the risks of it happening to them. I began to see infertility as an epidemic that no one was talking about.

Most of my friends were trying to get pregnant around the same time, and they knew as much, or as little, about their fertility as I knew about mine. It wasn't really a topic of conversation.

Like a lot of them, I'd spent my twenties trying to avoid getting pregnant. I did not feel I had the financial security, let alone the maturity, to become a parent in my twenties. I wanted to finish law school and start my career. More than anything, I wanted a secure relationship before having a child. Had I been better informed, I probably wouldn't have started much earlier than I did, but David and I would definitely have approached the initial years of trying very differently.

I don't exactly know how I had formed my impression of infertility treatment, but it was clearly not from a medical textbook. I thought a fertility doctor gave you some injections with a giant hormone-filled needle to jump start your ovaries, and then sent you back home to make a baby. That is not what happens. Rather, my fertility clinic became like a second home.

I chose a fertility clinic near my office and quickly learned how to get in and out within a couple of hours while trying to maintain a normal work life. I showed up at the front door of the clinic at 6:55 most mornings and stood outside with a handful of women in the cold and in the dark so that I could be one of the first people through the door when it opened. I'd rush out of the elevator to the reception desk to get my name on different clipboards, one for bloodwork, one for an ultrasound, and one to see the doctor. When I was undergoing a procedure, I was there almost daily for a month.

I started my days in a hospital gown, my feet holstered in oven mitts, with a technician using a medical tool on me that looked and felt suspiciously like a curling iron. It is amazing that something so invasive can be something you just get used to.

By 8 a.m., there were dozens of women waiting, so if you weren't in early, you were in for a very long wait. Privacy was impossible. Each time your name was called, it was shouted across the waiting room: "Alex . . . Alex Johnston!!"

Signs posted around the waiting room requested that you change into a hospital gown when you arrived to make the daily ultrasound process efficient. Less than half the women did this but I have a soft spot for rules, so I dutifully changed. It felt undignified wandering around the clinic in my undergarments every morning, but I wanted to do my part in helping the place to run smoothly. One day the fire alarm went off just as I was having my blood drawn. I was ushered out of the clinic, with all of the other women. As I walked down the internal staircase, realizing that I was about to stand on a street corner in a hospital gown in the middle of the morning rush hour, a block away from my office and certain to meet my colleagues as they poured out of the subway, I vowed that I would keep my pants on as long as possible going forward.

Eventually the signs were phased out. It seemed that even the clinic realized that the gowns, while efficient, were unnecessarily depersonalizing and demoralizing.

The waiting room was almost entirely women. No matter who had the fertility issues, it was women who went through the medical procedures because they were the ones who ultimately needed to get pregnant. Early on, David would come to try to be supportive but eventually, other than the times when he needed to provide a sperm sample, he got on with his day. The clinic itself wasn't designed for men. When we started, the waiting area was standing room only and the sample room, where men went to produce their sample, did double duty as a utility closet.

When you go to a clinic almost every day for five years, you run into people you know. I didn't want to talk and neither did they. We usually acknowledged each other with a nod and then left each other alone. There was a provincial cabinet minister who was going through treatments at the same time as me. We had worked together in government and she didn't like me very much. One morning she walked up to me in the waiting room and handed me her newspaper as she was leaving. This felt to me like her way of acknowledging that, whatever our professional differences may have been, we both knew how hard this experience was.

When women left the clinic each morning to rejoin the outside world, few people would know what we were experiencing. But the battle scars were visible to us. I watched many people cycle through the clinic over the years. I would often watch their spirits go from where I started, full of confidence that with a little help they would quickly be on the other side of infertility, to a more subdued place, understanding that the destination was far from certain. One day they would just stop showing up. I didn't know if they were successful and had moved on to an obstetrician or if they had given up.

As I sat in the waiting room, morning after morning, I realized that I had joined a club that I never wanted to be a part of. I had internalized the many stereotypes that applied to infertile women, never imagining that it would happen to me. I had assumed I would be like my mother, even though I was starting my family almost a decade later than she had started hers. I couldn't help but feel that my ignorance had put me in that waiting room.

I wanted to say to other women, "Do as I say, not as I do".

CHAPTER TWO

You Think You've Hit Rock Bottom, But Haven't

ASKED MY FERTILITY DOCTOR early on to advise me like I was her daughter. She said that if I was her daughter, she would tell me to move forward aggressively. If I wanted the possibility of having a child, I had no time to lose.

Each month David and I braced for bad news with failed cycle after failed cycle. I often thought, "This has to be rock bottom," but just when we thought things couldn't get worse, they always did.

As the failures racked up, I found myself in conversations with people who hadn't had any trouble getting pregnant, trying to figure out what they were doing right and what I was doing wrong, as if it were my fault. People would ask if maybe I thought I was exercising too much, or my job as a lawyer was too stressful. They wondered if I was eating the right foods or taking the right vitamins. All of it was well-intentioned but the implication was that I had to be doing something wrong for this to be happening to me. I knew women who smoked, who drank, who did hard drugs, and who still managed to get pregnant. My own situation was just the luck of the draw. My ovaries were simply depleting faster than the average woman my age.

In our first year at our fertility clinic we exhausted the recommended treatment path. This included up to four cycles of artificial insemination (IUI), where the doctor inserted sperm directly into my uterus with a catheter. My doctor and I used to joke that romance was highly overrated. I would lie still for fifteen minutes after the procedure and then hop off the gurney and head straight to work. IUI was, and is, a commonly used approach to treating infertility. The procedure cost about $400 per cycle. For an additional $80 I would take the drug Clomid, a small pill, administered orally, which helped my body produce multiple eggs, increasing my chances of conception. This approach was relatively inexpensive, but it significantly increased the odds of having multiples (twins or triplets), with much higher health risks and complications for mothers and babies.

When IUI didn't work we moved to the recommended four cycles of IVF, a far more expensive approach to treating infertility.

An ultrasound technician once told me that the waiting room in my fertility clinic was filled with professional women like me: doctors, lawyers, and businesswomen, because we waited too long to have children. I told her that it was filled with women like me because we were the only people who could afford to get help.

Unless you are fortunate enough to live in a country that covers fertility treatments or work for a company that provides good health benefits around fertility (and few do), the safest and best treatments, like IVF, are beyond the reach of most people. IVF costs upwards of $10,000 per cycle and several cycles are often needed to achieve a pregnancy. The drugs that accompany IVF can cost that much as well. For people struggling with infertility, the main barrier preventing many of them from having a child is often money.

IVF required daily doctors' visits. I injected hormones into my stomach each morning and evening to stimulate the production of multiple eggs. After a couple of weeks, when the eggs were mature, it was showtime.

The IVF procedure room at my clinic was connected to the laboratory, which is where a lot of the delicate work was done to grow the embryos. I would lie on a gurney, pumped full of sedatives, and my doctor would retrieve eggs from my ovaries. She would open up a window connecting the two rooms and carefully transfer the small tube containing the eggs to the embryologist. The eggs would be inseminated in a laboratory and the resulting embryos would grow in a petri dish. Three days later I would be back on the same gurney. The window would open. The embryologist would confirm our names to ensure the embryos were ours. Then she would put them under a microscope and give them a grade, letting us know their quality, right before she handed them in a tiny plastic tube to our doctor for the transfer. I would hold my breath before she graded them, but they were usually very good. We would marvel at the beauty of these little blob-like dots on the overhead screen. I would wonder, each time, how those little works of art could fail to grow to become a baby. This time had to be it.

But wherever those embryos went, they certainly didn't stick around my uterus long enough to register a pregnancy.

At my age, each round of IVF had a roughly 25% success rate. If you weren't successful after four cycles, then your odds of conceiving were very low.

After four unsuccessful tries, we had come to the first of what we didn't yet know would be many forks in the road, with nothing to show for our efforts except a thick medical file. We needed to make decisions around how to move forward. David was literally speechless by this point. He didn't seem angry. He just seemed overcome. I wondered if this might be it for him.

There were lots of online message boards discussing the pros and cons of continuing at this stage. People talked about coming to terms with the fact that they would not have a child. Some shared testimonials around how liberating it felt once they stopped trying: no more medical appointments and procedures, less stress, more travel, more money to do things like renovate their kitchen. None of these pros resonated with me.

I told David that I did not know how I was going to get there, but I was going the distance. I was open to different ways of becoming a parent including adoption or continuing fertility treatments but, with or without him, I was moving forward. I sat in a coffee shop with a friend one day sobbing. I did not know if or how my marriage would survive.

Our home felt like the loneliest place in the world. Ever since David and I met in university, our house had always been a mecca for friends. People often stayed in our home and ate at our table. Now we didn't invite anyone over anymore.

The hardest night of the year was probably Halloween, which seemed to have been designed to torture people who can't have children. Hundreds of kids in our neighbourhood would ring our doorbell with their little costumes and bags. I remember two young sisters bundled up in their beaten-up winter jackets and homemade toques trundling up our incredibly steep stairs one Halloween. I asked them what they were dressed as. They said princesses. I wanted to hug them. I just wanted one of those princesses to be mine.

Our loneliness was palpable. My mom emailed at one point to say that she wanted to get me a hairless, non-barking dog so that we would have another living creature in the house. I told her that sounded more like a goldfish. I really just wanted a child.

And, it turns out, David did, too.

David and I are both lawyers. We are pragmatic people and operate in a world of facts. We didn't know if our inability to conceive was an egg quality issue or if my body just couldn't carry a child.

We knew that if we wanted to become parents, we needed to change our approach. If my eggs were the issue, perhaps a donor egg was needed. We discussed different possibilities and decided that we would ask my youngest sister Sam to be our egg donor. When I asked her, she did not hesitate for a second. She was single and nowhere near thinking about pregnancy for herself. She was in the process of doing her PhD at Harvard. I knew this was not what she would have imagined doing in her twenties. But she loves me, and I love her. She wanted me to become a mother. She also ruined my favourite sweater when she was a teenager, so she sort of owed me.

David and I decided to try one last IVF with Sam. She flew into Toronto from Boston to live with us for a month while we went through an IVF cycle together. It turns out that she is afraid of needles and there were many a day, so I administered those for her. She describes me as a cross between Nurse Ratchet in *One Flew Over the Cuckoo's Nest* and Mr. Bean. I would characterize my nursing skills in more flattering terms, but the bottom line was I got the job done.

We synched up our bodies through an IVF cycle using her twenty-eight-year-old eggs and my thirty-four-year-old body. We transferred two embryos. I was optimistic that this would be it.

When I went for the pregnancy blood test after two weeks, there was not even a hint of a pregnancy. It seemed like my uterus just wasn't a hospitable place for a baby.

We were at another fork in the road.

* * *

I had heard a bit about surrogacy, but it was unusual enough back in 2005 that when I first raised the possibility with my fertility doctor, she asked me if David needed to have intercourse with the surrogate. I explained that would not be necessary.

At one point early in our journey, I was contacted by someone from National Geographic who had seen my profile on a website for people looking for surrogates. She was doing research on IVF and medical tourism and wondered if David and I would consider working with a surrogate and fertility clinic in India. Our treatment would be paid for, and we would be part of the research and story she was developing. It was significantly less expensive to do what we wanted to do in countries like India, but we did not know enough about the quality of the medical care, the laws around surrogacy, or the methods used to recruit surrogates to feel comfortable pursuing this option. Still, it spoke to the rise of infertility as a lucrative commercial area for many countries. After our years of navigating infertility, I became aware that if I had money, I could pretty much go anywhere in the world to set up a surrogacy arrangement that suited me.

I knew only one person who had used a surrogate mother to have her children and she knew a couple who had also worked with a surrogate. She reached out to them and they connected us to their surrogate. She was married, a stay-at-home mother of two boys. Like many people pursuing surrogacy for the first time, I couldn't fully understand how, at the end of the process, a surrogate wouldn't want to keep my baby. Doing this with someone who had done it before, and who knew what they were getting into, was important to me. When I went to her house for our first meeting, her boys were there. They were lovely. It was clear that she was a caring mother, which gave me confidence that she would care for my child in the same way that she cared for her own. She was also healthy and attractive, which made me feel that she took good care of herself.

Her home was on a cul-de-sac in a subdivision of a small Ontario town about two hours from my home. It was modest but well-maintained and seemed like a great place for her boys to grow up. She made a point of telling me that she and her husband had worked hard for everything that they had. Nothing had been given to them. I felt that she took pride in telling me this. I respected her attitude. I came from a comfortable background, but my parents faced difficult hardships in their own childhoods. They had built, together, from very little, the pretty spectacular life that my sisters and I grew up in.

She was clearly a determined person and she seemed determined to make me a mother. I liked her. We entered into a surrogacy agreement with her shortly after that first meeting.

It was the autumn of 2005, two and a half years after we first started trying to have children. I was working for the Premier of Ontario, Dalton McGuinty, managing his team of senior policy advisors, when our lawyer drafted our first surrogacy agreement.

It was legal in Canada to be a surrogate but commercial surrogacy, where the surrogate mother could profit from the pregnancy, was illegal. The law allowed for the reimbursement of reasonable expenses to a surrogate, but these weren't defined. The standard and legally accepted practice that had developed between surrogates and intended parents was to include a payment schedule in the surrogacy contract to cover expenses on a monthly basis, up to twenty thousand dollars over the course of the pregnancy.

The restrictions on commercial surrogacy inadvertently created a form of black market. Many experienced Canadian surrogates wanted approximately $5,000 to $10,000 more than was legally permitted in Canada, and they knew that they could get it if they worked with people in other countries. This meant that some Canadians entered into side agreements with their surrogates to supplement their legal contract. It seemed a reasonable amount of money to me, and it struck me as perverse that Canadian laws could turn otherwise law-abiding people into criminals so they could have a child. The penalties for breaking these laws included, then as now, financial penalties and jail time.

Our lawyer strongly cautioned us against entering into a side-agreement. She felt that I would be a very appealing test case for a first prosecution under the laws, given my job with the premier. With our luck up to that point, I thought how ironic it would be if we were finally able to have a baby and wound up in prison.

In August, just over a year since we had started fertility treatments, we tried our first IVF with a surrogate to see if this was the solution to our fertility issues. I took hormone injections to prepare for an egg retrieval. But this time I wasn't carrying. Our surrogate followed a protocol of progesterone supplements to prepare her uterus for an embryo transfer. She came to Toronto for the transfer and was confident from the get-go that she would become pregnant. She may have done home tests following the transfer, but she kept those results to herself. She told me that she always knew. When we got the official results at the two-week mark, she was, as she had anticipated, pregnant.

I couldn't believe it was this easy and wished we had moved to surrogacy earlier. We went to New York City to visit friends and splurged on tickets to see the tennis U.S. Open at Flushing Meadows. I remember walking to the top of the stands, scanning the beautiful skyline and feeling a lightness of being that is atypical for me. I'm a pretty wired person. David and I had been knocked down the previous few years, but it felt like things were looking up.

I called our surrogate to check on her. She was feeling good but told me that she had received the results from the second set of pregnancy blood tests that my clinic had done as part of monitoring the pregnancy. The nurse who had called her said the hormone levels were a bit lower than they wanted to see at this stage. Our surrogate wasn't concerned. She still felt very pregnant. I called our fertility specialist to check in. She told me the blood results weren't great but that she was "cautiously optimistic." I did not yet know that those words were code for, "things are going south, brace yourself for bad news."

Ten days later, our surrogate miscarried at six weeks.

We tried again a couple of months later in December 2005. Our surrogate liked to receive the information directly from the clinic and then she would call us. My fertility specialist wanted to make sure I was fine with that, and I was. It was my baby, but it was her body and I could tell that it was important for our surrogate to be able to share the news with us herself. I knew roughly when she was getting the results. I was driving to a meeting in a heavy snowfall, trying to focus on the road and not let my mind wander, when my phone rang. I pulled over and held my breath. She was pregnant. The blood test results were excellent, suggesting the pregnancy was very viable. I was delighted. The greatest gift anyone could give us was a child. It was right before Christmas.

My fertility doctor followed the pregnancy until just after the three-month mark. Before she relinquished care to an obstetrician, we did a 3-D ultrasound. It was mind-blowing. It was like looking at your baby through a window. We marvelled that we could see its facial features so clearly. We learned that we were expecting a girl. This baby felt as real as anything I had ever experienced.

Because of surrogacy's uniqueness, I was often on the receiving end of questions from friends, colleagues, and acquaintances trying to understand how it worked and why I was doing it. I was often asked by other mothers whether I was worried I would not be able to love my child because I wasn't carrying. I would simply ask if they had worried that their child's father would not be able to love their child. Those fathers hadn't carried their child either, after all.

Because of the ban on commercial surrogacy, there was a lingering perception that surrogacy itself was a little bit "wrong." Even people who were totally uninformed about surrogacy were often quick to offer an opinion. My mother was accosted by an acquaintance in the grocery store of her small community. The woman had heard about my surrogacy and asked my mother how she could condone her daughter doing something illegal to have a child. She spoke about me like I was a human trafficker. I explained to my mom that it wasn't illegal, it was just unusual. I also tried to persuade her to cough up the woman's address so I could leave a dead squirrel on her porch.

Our surrogate wanted to work with the doctor at her regional hospital who had supervised her pregnancies with her sons. I was fine with that, although it was clear when I went to the first appointment with her that the doctor did not have any experience with surrogacy. When I attended appointments, the doctor frequently reminded me that our surrogate was the patient and that I had no right to any information about the baby or the pregnancy. Even though David and I were in equal parts the genetic parents, we were treated very differently. At medical appointments, he was treated like the father. I was a third wheel. Both the doctor and the hospital struggled to understand my place in all of this.

I believe mine was the first surrogate pregnancy the hospital had managed. I began meeting with a hospital administrator early on in the pregnancy to work out a plan for the birth. I would be allowed in the delivery room, but David would have all decision-making rights following the birth, reinforcing my second-class status. As frustrating and, at times, hurtful as this was, these felt like minor issues given the very long journey it had taken to get to a place where we were having actual conversations about a real child.

A healthy baby's heartbeat in utero is a beautiful sound. We had a medical appointment on a Sunday, the day before the due date. I sat there listening to her heartbeat, beating like a drum, strong and rhythmic, knowing this was our last appointment. Everything looked good but there were no signs of labour. An induction date was scheduled for the Wednesday if nothing had happened by then.

I felt calm and happy. My child was in no rush to meet the world but in the next seventy-two hours, I was going to become a mother.

I drove my surrogate home and arranged to pick her up early on the morning of the induction and drive her to the hospital. The baby's room was set up. I was winding down work. That Monday, someone in the premier's office had unexpectedly sent out an email to a very broad group of colleagues letting people know that I was going on maternity leave. I was only going to be gone a few months since David and I were splitting our parental leave. Of course, outside of my immediate colleagues, not a lot of people at work knew I was expecting a child because I wasn't pregnant. I had planned to describe it as a leave of absence so that I wouldn't have to answer all of the questions that would inevitably come along with a surrogacy. Now hundreds of people knew. I spent my last week at work fielding questions in meeting rooms, elevators and stairwells about adoption, which is what most people assumed we were doing. When I would tell them that we were expecting a child through surrogacy, most people just stared at me blankly. They didn't quite know what it was or what to say.

I was happy to attend one last work event before all hell broke loose in my house with a newborn. It was an end-of-summer BBQ hosted by the premier for his senior staff. He had an idea of how gruelling the last couple of years had been for David and I; like all of my colleagues, he was happy for us. He is a lawyer by training and a curious person by nature. I had forgotten that he had studied biology before law and there was no one in the office more interested in surrogacy than him. It was all I could do not to draw a diagram on a white board in his office, explaining the mechanics. His questions always felt kind and supportive and true to who he was, a fifty something-year-old man trying to understand advances in reproductive medicine that were very foreign to him.

In the weeks leading up to the birth, someone said to me that when I reached the other side of all of this, the process of getting there would feel like a distant memory. That pretty much summed up how I felt going to bed that night. I felt nothing but gratitude. For David, for our surrogate, for modern medicine. For my life.

I slept well that night.

That next afternoon, the day before the scheduled induction date, my surrogate called me at work to let me know that labour had started spontaneously. Her water had not broken but contractions had begun. She was in contact with a nurse at the hospital by phone who had advised her to stay home until her contractions were closer together. In retrospect, this was incredibly bad advice.

An hour later, she called again to let me know that things were progressing quickly. The baby was very active and her neighbour was driving her to the hospital. I called David to let him know that we needed to get to the hospital as soon as possible. We met at home to get our car and the baby's bag that we had prepared for the birth. I had also put together a bag of fun things, like magazines, cards, and snacks for me and our surrogate to bide the time while we waited for labour to start. It felt like that bag probably wasn't going to be needed at this point.

I had done the ninety-minutes from our house to the hospital many times but doing it in rush hour traffic felt like an eternity. I called my sister Sharon, a doctor, and told her what was going on. She reassured me that one way or another, babies come out. She and I speculated that the baby might be born by the time I got to the hospital.

We arrived at the hospital and parked the car. As I walked through the parking lot, I realized I had sandals on. I ran back to the car to change into sneakers. This felt like the most important moment in my life and I wanted my feet to be firmly grounded. We struggled to find our surrogate inside the hospital. Her neighbour had kindly called to let me know that she had dropped her off at the ER and reassured me that she just needed a good epidural. When we were finally directed from the ER to obstetrics, I gave the nurse at the front desk our names. She was terse and asked how we were connected to our surrogate. I told her that we were the parents and were there for the birth of our daughter. She sent us to a waiting room down an empty hallway and told us the doctor would come see us. I assumed things were too far along by that point for me to be in the delivery room.

After sitting for what felt like a very long time, I looked around the room and realized it was eerily empty. I had been to the obstetrics area many times before. I had always waited in a crowded room full of well-worn chairs and magazines. This room didn't have a trace of anyone ever having set foot in it before us. The décor was dated but the furniture was pristine. The room was spotless and sterile. It is the only room I have ever been in that smelled like nothing. There were no signs of life, not a plant, not a garbage can or a crumb of food. I asked David to go see what was going on. He stepped out of the room and immediately looked back at me. He told me a group of people were walking down the hallway towards us. My heart quickened. I thought they were coming to tell us that I couldn't be in the delivery room. I wasn't going to argue. I just wanted to meet my daughter.

The doctor started telling us something about our surrogate arriving at the hospital in advanced labour. There was no fetal heartbeat when she arrived. He told us that they had tried unsuccessfully to resuscitate the baby but that she was stillborn.

The information was coming at me like bullets. I just stood there wide eyed, not sure that this was real. An older Scottish nurse was there; she had been at my last few medical appointments with my surrogate and had seemed truly happy for me. She tried to hug me. I pushed her away instinctively even though I understood that she had nothing to do with what was going on. I couldn't process the information I had just received, let alone be comforted. Every word felt like a body blow. I was just trying to stay standing. I wanted to place my fingers on the doctor's lips and tell him to stop speaking. I could not believe this was happening. I could not believe this was my life.

The doctor told us that the attending doctor who delivered our baby was just about to go off shift. He would be leaving soon so if we wanted more information then we needed to see him now. He came and explained to us that our daughter had passed her first stool, her meconium, in utero during labour; it is something that usually happens after a baby is born, but can happen earlier when babies are in distress. She had suffocated inhaling it.

It was a traumatic delivery and they were cleaning her up so that we could see her. I called Sharon to let her know the baby had died in labour on the way to the hospital. I held it together enough to transfer the information that needed to be transferred. I told her the name of the hospital. I said that I needed her to take care of whatever needed to be done to claim the body and to let the rest of our family know. It was the most painful conversation we had ever had. I am sure her heart was breaking but she took over all of the things I could not face that night.

I told David that I didn't know how I was going to get through this but that if we were going to get through it together, we would have to carry each other. I had reached my breaking point.

I checked on our surrogate to make sure that she was okay. I sat on the edge of her bed in the recovery room and we just cried. Whatever had transpired in those few hours, I knew that she needed my reassurance. She would have her own difficult path towards healing.

Then David and I went to spend time with our daughter. A colleague had been through something similar a few years earlier. I attended the funeral for her first child, a baby boy who was stillborn at full term. Her voice guided me through my steps that night, telling me that she had named him, held him, and honoured him with a proper burial.

We did all of those things. We named our daughter Sam, my favourite name for a girl. We held her for a few hours in the hospital room where they brought her to us. We took pictures cradling her in our arms. A very kind local photographer had a standing offer with the hospital to discreetly take pictures when a baby was stillborn if the parents wanted it. He charged nothing for this and, while I don't remember anyone being in the room that night, I cherish the pictures he took of us holding Sam swaddled in a blanket as if she was just sleeping. Her face is still, and her lips are blue, but you can see what a lovely, healthy baby girl she would have been.

The photos are all we have. They are profoundly beautiful and heartbreaking. They captured the love for our daughter and the depth of our sorrow.

CHAPTER THREE

Sorrow

W E STOOD OUTSIDE THE HOSPITAL late that night not sure what would happen next but knowing that we had to go home. I can still feel the warm summer breeze on my face as we walked to our car. It was August 29, two days before our fourth wedding anniversary. We drove in silence. I don't know what David was thinking but I was trying to grasp what specifically had changed in that short period. We had arrived at the hospital without a child and we were going home without a child. Why did it feel like someone had ripped my heart out of my body?

When I posed that question to someone the next day she said, "Because you became parents last night."

My own parents lived on a beautiful horse farm in the middle of a small Mennonite farming community outside of Kitchener-Waterloo, Ontario. Their neighbours were salt of the earth, horse-and-buggy people. We had exchanged marriage vows on the farm, under an oak tree, surrounded by friends and family, on a beautiful August day. Four years later we were planning a funeral service there for our daughter. I didn't know how to bury a baby. I told my family to tell our friends they didn't need to come. It seemed like it was something you did quietly with your family. Our friends ignored me. Many of them drove or flew from cities near and far away. They piled out of cars and taxis and showed up on our doorstep in Toronto. I looked out my window two days after we lost Sam and two of my closest friends from Montreal, Mary and Timon, were getting out of their car. A month earlier we had been in Maine together with their two young children, celebrating the imminent arrival of Sam. I walked out of the house and just let them hold me.

I hadn't known what I needed but our friends knew we needed them. They dismantled the baby's room and sent our stuff to people who needed it. They sat with us, often in silence, so we wouldn't be alone. They bought groceries and made food. And they came together, on a beautiful end of summer day, at my parents' farm, to help us honour Sam. I can hardly remember who was there, but I saw a sea of faces and I knew they wanted us to know that we were loved. David could not speak so I prepared some words about the child we would never have a chance to know or to raise. I don't remember what I said, but I do remember facing the wind, looking across the fields full of hay with the sun beating down on us. I thought of how unfair this was to Sam. I thought of how much the hospital had struggled to understand my role but that day my role in Sam's life couldn't have been clearer. You needed to look no further than the two broken people carrying her small coffin to the hearse to know who Sam's parents were.

As our new reality settled in over the next few weeks, I chain-smoked and relied on sleeping pills to have a few hours each night away from the pain. These things held me up like crutches. I was a shell of the person I had been just a few days earlier.

We had dinner early on with my colleague and her husband whose son was stillborn. By then they were parents to three more children. They were and are caring people, and they tried to help us understand that we would be out of this terrible place at some point. But there was a way they looked at us that I found unsettling.

I couldn't pinpoint what it was. I understood much later that what their eyes conveyed was knowledge. They had experienced their own trauma and their compassion came from a place of deep understanding. They knew that we hadn't yet fully grasped how truly harrowing the journey to the other side would be.

As the shock wore off, David and I entered a very dark place. Most of our friends either had or were having babies and we couldn't be around babies. We have no end of loving people in our life but in grief people have their own feelings and needs they want met. We couldn't be the people to meet those needs. Many people want to love you the way they want you to be loved, which isn't necessarily the way you need to be loved.

For the most part, time and space were what we needed most. I was the maid of honour for a close friend a few weeks before Sam died. Then she got pregnant a few months after her wedding, and we became estranged. I just stopped returning her calls and emails. When I showed up on her doorstep almost two years later, I started to apologize. She stopped me mid-sentence and said, "You don't need to apologize, I'm just so glad you're here." It felt like the most loving gesture a friend could have offered me.

My sister Sharon, who helped carry me through the first few months after we lost Sam, gave birth to twins the following July. We live in different cities and I didn't see her during her pregnancy. It was a difficult birth and my mom was with her that night. My dad stayed over at my home in Toronto. He let me know, as soon as he knew, that my sister and the babies were doing fine, which was important to me. Then he said nothing else about it. He loved us both so much. I imagine his heart was split in two experiencing these two very different realities with his daughters.

I wasn't able to meet my niece and nephew, who I love like my own kids today, until they were over a year old. I used to joke with my sister that if I went to meet them there was a thirty percent chance that I would throw them in my car and just keep driving. I tried to visit a few times but, the truth was, I didn't want to hold another baby until I held my own again.

In this fragile state, David and I disconnected from most of our social community. We both went back to work after six weeks to get away from our loneliness and try to have a focus beyond our grief. I remember two things from that first day back at work. I chose a quiet time to arrive that morning so that I could go discreetly to my office and wouldn't be overwhelmed by people. I entered the building and walked to the elevator with no one around. Just as I got into the elevator, the husband of one of my closest work friends got in as well. His wife had delivered their daughter a few days before Sam was born and he was just coming back to work from his paternity leave. We looked at each other and rode in silence as that difficult coincidence hung in the air. There really was nothing to say.

At the end of that first day, I closed my door and sat in my dark office watching the sun go down behind the parliament building across the street, tears streaming down my face. I didn't know how I was going to do this. I didn't want to be at work, and I didn't want to be at home. There was nowhere I wanted to be. There was a knock on the door and the premier's executive assistant asked to come in. I told her it wasn't a good time, but she was insistent. When I opened the door, she said the premier wanted to come and see me. He is a father of four children and, as we sat in my office, he said that he had often thought of how helpless my own parents must feel not being able to protect me. He had been at Sam's funeral and had spent much of the time speaking with them. He told me to pace myself and to rely on my work family to rally around me. I nodded knowing that I would need them to help me get through this.

I have often been asked whether having another child at home would have been helpful. I don't know. I remember the first time I heard President Joe Biden speak about losing his wife and daughter in a car accident. The interviewer asked him if he had wanted to die. I expected him to give some political answer about how his faith carried him. Instead, he was honest. He said that he did want to die but that he had two little boys to care for who had lost their mother and sister. He got up every morning for them. I was grateful for his candour.

As much as I loved my husband, it felt like I had no one to get up for. I did want to die, every day, for a long time. The grief didn't just break my heart, it almost broke my brain. I couldn't make sense of what had happened. We came within thirty minutes of meeting our daughter alive and being able to bring her home from the hospital. We ended up on a very different path from the one we had expected to be on.

There were nights that I just walked around our neighbourhood trying to focus on taking one breath at a time so that I could make it through the evening until I went to bed. Then I would do it all over again the next day. I made a conscious choice to try to get up each morning and make it through that particular day unsure if I would be able to make it through the next. I took comfort in feeling like that choice gave me some degree of control in all of this.

I knew I had been very lucky up until that point. I didn't feel like I deserved to avoid suffering. But I was overcome by the relentless and excruciating reality of the pain.

The grieving process is unique for each person. For me, it was an endless, full body, all-consuming experience. There was no relief. I felt like I was drowning every moment of every day. I figured one day I would just sink.

Someone suggested I go on anti-depressants. I would have gratefully accepted any help, but I felt that this experience was very different from depression.

I read books on the various stages of grief but there was nothing linear about my process. The stages whirled around me every day like a hurricane.

I have a very close friend who lost her brother about a year after we lost Sam. He was a police officer and father of a young daughter, and he was shot and killed on the job. I did not know her well when it happened, but it was a news story and the moment I heard about it I felt such profound sadness for her. I knew that the life she knew was gone. As she grieved her loss, someone suggested she reach out to me. Our experiences were dissimilar, but we connected around our shared understanding of grief and sorrow. We held each other up and joked about some of the crazy things people did and said to try to make us feel better. Sometimes we reflected on the fact that we knew other people had it worse and wondered how they survived their grief when we could barely survive ours.

My friend had joined a bereavement group for young women when her brother died. One of the group members had lost her parents and her sister in a car accident. When my friend told me about her, I remembered having read about it in the newspaper and wondering, at the time, whether she would ever be okay.

Similarly, I was driving one day while listening to a woman on the radio discuss the Rwandan genocide. She was so thoughtful and well-spoken that I assumed she was an academic. It turned out that she was a survivor and had lost her entire family. I could not believe that she was still standing and yet, here she was, using her experience to educate others.

Even with this perspective, your own grief is yours alone.

There were many days when mine felt too much to carry.

David and I have loved each other since we met at university. I couldn't imagine that this was how our story would end but it was clear that we had finally hit rock bottom. Our beautiful conversation in Italy, where we decided to start our family, had led us to this unexpectedly terrible place.

We were in our mid-thirties and having a baby would, at best, require a small army. At worst, it would not happen at all. Infertility had made me as helpless as I have ever been, totally dependent on others to do what David and I wanted more than anything: to have a child.

I knew that to get through this, I had to make choices that would not just give me comfort but would give me strength. I cut out the cigarettes and stopped the sleeping pills.

I realized the only way through this, for me, was to become a parent again.

CHAPTER FOUR

Life After Death

L IFE IS FULL OF EXPERIENCES that help you grow and mature. Some of these are gentle. Some are not. Infertility felt altogether different. It felt like an experience you simply survive.

Losing Sam almost broke me. It broke parts of me that I now know, with the benefit of time, can't be put back together. I am a happy person, so it is hard to put a finger on what it is that I lost. I imagine it is different for each person but there is a childhood memory that captures it best for me.

When I was nine, my parents moved our family from London, Ontario to Montreal, Quebec for my dad's work. We were moving for him to become the principal of McGill University. At the time, Quebec was on the cusp of a referendum to vote on whether to separate from the rest of Canada. If we weren't the only English Canadian family that moved to Quebec that year, then we certainly were one of the few. My parents put me and my sisters in French school right away.

Politics in Quebec were volatile. At times, as recently as the 1970s, they had been violent. Because of this, there was some concern that our family would be targeted given our connection to a prominent English institution. The safety concerns meant that we had to be driven to our very mixed-income school by a professional driver employed by McGill. His name was Mike and he was incredibly kind to us. I used to beg him to drop me off at least a block away, so kids didn't know we were being chauffeured. He empathized but said he had to get us safely to school before he could leave us.

Being a unilingual anglophone in a French school during the referendum was not an easy starting point for fitting in, let alone for making friends. I spent most of my days that first year fending off the bullies that bothered me and my younger sisters. Shortly after starting, a kid spat in my eye during recess one day. I asked another student to help me tell the recess monitor what had happened. The monitor, Soeur Juliette, was a Catholic nun who was notoriously strict but also fair. I marched up to her and explained, with my limited French and the help of the other student, what had occurred. When I finished, I expected her to go find the kid. Instead, she chastised me and sent me away. The incident baffled me until I understood, much later on, as my French improved, that my "translator" had given me the French word for "fart" instead of "spit." I had explained to Soeur Juliette that someone had farted in my eye.

It was a rough time for me and my sisters, which we now simply refer to as "character building".

A few years after the move, my parents took us to France one summer to better appreciate what learning a new language and culture had given us. It brought all of our effort home in a very real way. One day we were picnicking off the road somewhere beautiful. I wandered off for a walk. I ended up in a forest with the sun beaming through the trees, the sound of a stream in the background, and a warm and gentle breeze weaving its way through the forest. It felt almost too good to be real. I started dancing alone in the woods. I don't know how long I danced but, at some point, I realized that a couple of my sisters were watching me from behind a boulder. By the way they were laughing, they clearly had been watching me for some time. Anyone with siblings can appreciate that the only thing worse than getting caught dancing alone in a French forest is spending the next month in a cramped car being ridiculed. But the feeling I had dancing in the forest has stayed with me always.

It was the first time I consciously remember feeling joy.

I danced through my teens, my twenties, and into my early thirties. When I moved from Montreal to Toronto after finishing law school and started practicing law, I still danced. I used to go to a drop-in dance jam called Sweat Your Prayers in a giant light-filled studio. Strangers would show up and dance it out for ninety minutes to a DJ-led rhythmic music compilation designed to get you in touch with your body, mind, and soul. I would inevitably start each time thinking that I had made a big mistake. I would find myself dancing beside a man, dressed as a woman, dancing like a swaying tree, a markedly different demographic from my professional world. I would think that I was too serious to let loose with a bunch of strangers. But, without fail, I'd be dancing within minutes. The world outside of that room would slip away and I would just dance.

If I could sum up in one sentence what infertility did to me, it snuffed the life out of that dancer. She is pretty much gone. She comes out at weddings occasionally.

* * *

Dancer or no dancer, I was intent on taking the steps to rebuild a full and happy life on the other side of infertility and losing Sam. I took good care of myself. I exercised and ate well. I got professional help for my mental health and shared with my therapist the saddest, darkest thoughts a human can share, thoughts that I couldn't share with anyone else. I reached out to others, friends, family members, colleagues and bosses, to ask for what I needed.

I was lucky to have access to all of the care that helped me get better. Many people don't have the supports that I had to make it to the other side of grief. When I see people struggling to live healthy and functional lives, I try not to judge. I wonder what broke them. I know they have their own backstories. I imagine that I could easily be in the same situation.

When Sam died, I was thirty-six years old, we were four years into infertility, and there was no easy path for David and I to become parents again.

We were open to adoption. My parents' family doctor had contacted them at one point about one of his patients, a university student, who was unexpectedly pregnant and considering placing the baby up for adoption. He wondered if we were interested in meeting with her. We let him know that we were. I imagined what a difficult and life-changing decision this must be for her. I thought how distraught I would have been at her age, navigating my choices. In the end she decided to keep her baby. It sounded like she felt that she had the family support that she needed to raise a child on her own. I was glad that she made a decision that felt right for her.

I had also watched my older sister, Deb, adopt two girls, now my two nieces, from Cali, Columbia. The arrival of her daughters Emma and Tea, the first two grandchildren for my parents, changed our family. They opened up our hearts to a very different kind of love, the kind reserved only for children. But I knew watching my sister navigate the adoption process that it came with its own set of battle scars. Constantly shifting international rules and regulations, long wait lists, home visits by social workers assessing my sister and her husband's fitness to parent, and an enormous amount of time and money were some of the challenges she faced through an eight-year process.

My desire to create a child together with the person I loved was deep. Surrogacy still felt like the right option for us. So, only weeks removed from the funeral, we started the process of finding another surrogate all over again.

We were grieving the loss of Sam profoundly. At the same time, as difficult as it felt, we knew it was important to take the steps to try and move our life forward and build our family.

Working with Sam's surrogate was not an option.

I checked on her a number of times that fall to make sure that she was recovering physically and emotionally. Eventually I needed to bring the relationship to a close. The main connection was this one traumatic experience. Our experience, as parents, was very different from hers.

David and I needed to grieve it alone.

People often asked me why a woman would want to carry another person's baby. I am far from an expert but, having worked with or screened many surrogates over the years, I'd say there are a number of factors. Most of the surrogates I encountered had their own children, they were from lower-middle to middle income backgrounds, they got pregnant easily, and enjoyed pregnancy. Typically, there was a combination of a financial and altruistic motivation.

I wanted our surrogates to have both. The financial motivation was important to me because I wanted them to have their own incentives. I didn't want them to be doing this just for us; I wanted them to be doing this for them. Given that the median family income in Canada is about $70,000 and in the U.S about $61,000, the income from a surrogacy can be significant for a family. Altruism is often an important secondary motivator: my surrogates clearly wanted to help us become parents. But if you remove the financial component, I believe that few women in Canada or the U.S. would become surrogates.

We were open to working with Canadian and U.S surrogates. I began interviewing, on the phone or in person, potential surrogates and they, in turn, interviewed me. They were screening me to make sure I was the kind of person they wanted to do this with and that my eggs were still viable enough that we were likely to achieve a pregnancy. My own long battle with infertility may have seemed daunting to some but the fact that we had worked with a surrogate who had become pregnant may have reassured others. One experienced surrogate I interviewed opted against working with us. We met at a McDonald's halfway between her home and mine, once. Following that meeting she chose another couple. Surrogates don't want to waste their time going down this road with someone if they didn't feel there was a high likelihood of success.

I was screening surrogates to assess their fertility potential and whether they seemed like someone I wanted carrying my child. I also wanted to ensure they had a support network that was comfortable with surrogacy to help them through the pregnancy.

We found our second surrogate, Michelle, in the U.S. through an online message board on a surrogacy website called SurroMomsOnline. At the time, it was an important online community and platform to help surrogates and intended parents find each other without having to pay an agency, whose fees could run upwards of $25,000.

In the U.S., unlike Canada, a surrogacy arrangement is a negotiated commercial contract. The financial component is a significant part of the negotiation. When we were doing this, there was a wide range in compensation based on the market. Surrogates in California were getting as much as $80,000 whereas surrogates located in the Northeast and Midwest, where we were looking, were typically getting somewhere between $25-30,000. Finding someone to carry our baby was more expensive in the U.S., but I liked the ability to freely negotiate a contract and pay our surrogate what felt like a fair amount for what she was undertaking. I wanted her to benefit from our relationship too.

Michelle lived in Indiana, and had five children of her own, between eight and twenty years old. She had been a traditional surrogate, where she carried and used her own eggs, once before with a couple who lived near her.

Clearly, she was very fertile, and we were keen to keep the process moving. I had done a few IVF cycles and froze embryos for a future sibling while we were expecting Sam. I felt confident that we had what we needed to make this happen. We tried five times over the next year with Michelle. She never got pregnant.

When I told Michelle that we were not going to try again with her, she was disappointed and angry. I understood her disappointment because she had her own set of financial and emotional expectations. In the absence of a pregnancy, most of these had not been met. For whatever reason, our embryos and her body were a bad match.

There was no point in continuing to try.

I began putting the pieces in place for one final act. This time, I was leaving no stone unturned.

CHAPTER FIVE

Starting Over

S HORTLY AFTER WE PARTED ways with Michelle, I met with my fertility doctor. David and I were closing in on five years of infertility and a not insignificant financial invest-ment. We had a miscarriage, a stillbirth, and a second unsuccessful surrogacy to show for it. A lot of our path had simply been terrible luck. Our doctor was too professional and experienced to make false promises like, "I'm going to make this happen." But we wanted to bring this chapter to a close and he wanted that for us as well.

It felt like I was planning a small military operation. My plan would involve David and me, with a backup egg donor, and one or possibly two surrogates.

The doctor asked the right questions when I presented it to him. Specifically, he wanted to make sure that we had thought through all relevant possibilities, including finding ourselves with more than one child. We talked it over and agreed that if that were to happen then David and I could manage.

I looked into his eyes and I told him the plane had been circling for too long. I needed him to land it. Someone needed to get pregnant.

I had used up all of our frozen embryos with Michelle. My body was hitting a wall. It seemed to be shutting down. I still planned to do IVF once I found a surrogate, but I called my sister Sharon to ask if she would consider being my egg donor if I needed that. My two youngest sisters, Sam and Jen, were getting ready to start their own families by then. Sharon had her twins and she was not planning on having any more children. She seemed, at that point, like the best family candidate. It didn't hurt that she had played varsity hockey at Harvard and finished at the top of her medical school class at Dartmouth.

Sharon is eighteen months younger than me. She is a family doctor married to an emergency room pediatrician. She is, and always has been, as dear to me as anyone in my life. She would pretty much say the same of me even though I vacuumed some of her hair off when she was six. To be fair, I thought that every vacuum cleaner attachment would have the same effect as the hose, transforming dirty hair into a ponytail. It turned out the attachment with the wheels gave us a very different result. You only make that mistake once.

She said that she had been waiting for me to ask. She was ready if I needed her. She said she was simply providing her DNA, which was similar to my DNA. I was not surprised by her answer, but I asked if she had discussed this with her husband. It was not a given that my brother-in-law, or anyone, for that matter, could get their heads around my request or my sister's decision. She said that he was on board. Given the close relationship I have with my brother-in-law today, his support for her decision, which would have implications for him and their two children if we were successful using her eggs, does not surprise me. But I didn't know him as well then.

She and I talked through a few important considerations like what kind of an attachment she imagined she might have to the child. She expected that she would have a special connection but thought she would have that anyway because of our own close relationship. I felt the same way. We both agreed that the child would likely be short and bossy.

Her only concern, which knowing her is not a shocker, was figuring out the scheduling and logistics. She could manage the medication and injections on her own with the help of a fertility clinic close to her home. But she would need to come to Toronto for an egg retrieval at my fertility clinic at some undetermined time. She wanted to manage the timing and travel in a way that would minimize the disruption for her kids, her husband, her patients, and her dog. She is, if nothing else, pragmatic.

That same week, out of the blue, I got a call at work from one of our closest friends, Chella. She said that she had decided at Sam's funeral that she would offer to be our surrogate, but she wanted her husband to be comfortable with the idea. He had told her the night before, just after the one-year anniversary of Sam's death, that he was. It still brings tears to my eyes thinking about the profound love that prompted her to make that call. I was then working around the clock at campaign headquarters, managing the policy team during an election. I was sitting at a cubicle jammed in a boardroom with twenty other people around me. I couldn't speak freely, and I was trying not to cry.

We talked later that night, agreeing that there were steps we needed to take to ensure she had fully considered this decision. There was no one that David and I would trust more with a baby than Chella. We understood the significance of her offer. I made appointments for her with a social worker and with my fertility doctor. The main take-away was exactly what she had expressed to me. She did not want to be pregnant again (she had her own three children) but she wanted more than anything for David and I to have our own family.

We tried once with Chella as our surrogate. She was travelling to New Zealand for a family trip the following year. We had a small window to make it happen before then. It was the only time in all of my years at my fertility clinic that they botched the procedure. There was a breakdown in communication between clinic staff during the cycle, which led to an error in administering my medication. When someone realized the error, I was rushed in for an emergency egg retrieval to get the eggs out before they spontaneously burst, leaving me with ovarian cysts that would take months to resolve. An otherwise successful cycle was a bust. The clinic reimbursed our money but the window of opportunity with Chella had closed.

* * *

It is draining to live in a perpetual state of pain and vulnerability. I was tired of being sad all the time. Aside from the practical value of what Chella and Sharon had offered, what they did made me feel less alone than I had in a long time. Just reaching over the divide between our personal world and the outside world made David and I feel so loved. We were no closer to a pregnancy but a weight had lifted.

The missing piece was a surrogate.

Meeting Debbie felt like a cross between a blind date and an important job interview. I wanted her to do a surrogacy with us, so I was conscious of putting my best foot forward. But I also wanted to find someone who was going to be as committed to getting to the other side as we were.

We met, for the first time, for coffee at a Tim Hortons half-way between Toronto, where I live, and the small Ontario town where she lives. She is quiet, shy, and a private person by nature. She is petite, strawberry blonde, blue-eyed, and freckled and we could have passed as sisters. I had suggested that we meet at her house, which would have given me a broader context in which to get to know her and potentially meet her husband and two young children, but it was clear that she did not want that.

I had found Debbie through a surrogacy matching service that helped surrogates and intended parents find each other. I had submitted a profile of David and I, so Debbie had some background information for our meeting. I am an extrovert and she is an introvert, but we developed an easy rapport. She struck me as a gentle and caring person. She had spent a great deal of time in hospitals with a husband who had serious health issues, including a benign, untreatable brain tumour and kidney failure. He had had a transplant by then but suffered from chronic health problems. I wondered, with everything she had going on, why she had made the decision to become a surrogate. She said that when she first read about surrogacy, she knew it was something that she wanted to do for herself. It seemed like an act of empowerment.

Her first surrogacy was twins, so I felt that she understood what she was in for. I told her that David and I might work with two surrogates simultaneously and wondered how she would feel if we did. Not all surrogates would agree. Many surrogates would not be comfortable knowing there might be another surrogate. She said that she would be fine with that. She was interested in doing a surrogacy with us but needed to wait a few months to fully recover physically from her previous surrogacy. It was the fall of 2007.

Near the end of our conversation, Debbie said that when she first read our profiles, which disclosed that we had already worked with a surrogate and lost our baby in labour and delivery, she remembered her sister sharing a similar story. Her sister was a nurse at the hospital where Sam was delivered. She was working the night that Sam had died. Debbie asked if I was that baby's mother. I was a bit startled by this coincidence and I confirmed that I was.

It was clear that her compassion was a significant motivator for her wanting to be a surrogate for me. I knew that I wanted to do this with her.

In January 2008, we entered into a surrogacy contract with Debbie. She got pregnant with our first IVF attempt in mid-March. We found out on David's fortieth birthday, April Fool's Day. It felt good but by then we approached any good news with caution.

The previous fall, just as we started putting the pieces in place with Debbie, we began exploring a second surrogacy. Our plan of attack had not changed. We wanted to do this with two experienced surrogates simultaneously, so we cast a wide net. We found our last surrogate, Diane, in Green Bay, Wisconsin through a U.S. agency that specialized in surrogacy.

Diane had been a surrogate twice before. She was transparent with me in our first telephone call that she had to bring her first set of parents to court. She had an emergency C-section because of an unexpected medical condition that arose during pregnancy. They refused to pay her full compensation. She successfully sued them in court to fulfill the remainder of her contract. I was impressed that she had stood up for herself. I also appreciated that she shared this information, which helped form my impression of her. She connected me to the mother from her second surrogacy as a reference. She was glowing in her description of Diane as a surrogate and also as a person.

Diane worked as a nurse's aide in a long-term care facility in Wisconsin. It was not an easy job, but she seemed genuinely interested in the residents and showed great care and compassion for them through the stories she told. She seemed straight-forward and very likeable.

At forty-five years old, she did not want to waste any time. She was interested in potentially doing another surrogacy after ours and the older you are, the harder it is to find people who will work with you. Women's eggs may be done by their forties, but many women can physically carry a baby for a long time after that. We lined things up quickly.

Diane took a flight to Toronto in November 2007 for our first IVF together. She had a passport, but she had never been outside the U.S. We worried that taking a random trip to Toronto, a city where she had no family and friends, was unusual enough that she would be pulled aside by border security and, that if she disclosed the real reason for her trip, she might not make it into the country. What we were about to do together was perfectly legal but rare. We agreed that she would say that her reason for coming to Toronto was to support a friend through infertility and that we had met through the international infertility community. That had the dual benefit of being both true and strategic. We speculated that once she started talking about "lady parts" a customs official would wave her through pretty quickly. We were right.

I picked her up outside the airport. We were meeting face to face for the first time. I don't remember all of the details, but I remember being shocked by how striking she is. Diane is a tall, brown-haired beauty. She is gregarious and big in stature and personality.

As different as Diane and Debbie were, their character and values were similar. They had both experienced challenges in their own lives and navigated these with strength and clarity. They never met but I always thought they would like each other if they did.

We chatted comfortably as we drove to my house. The plan was for Diane to stay at our house overnight and we would head to the fertility clinic the next day to do the IVF procedure. Diane isn't someone to get easily flustered but she was honest that she felt a bit out of her element. She was struck by how busy and intense the city was, even that late at night. I reassured her that it was a wonderful city and I felt very lucky to live there. When we got to my home, just before midnight, my street was cordoned off with police tape. There were police cars and lights all down the street. I rolled down the window to speak to one of the officers. He explained that there was a shoot-out a block from my house. Someone had been chased up the street and shot to death. I honestly thought Diane would just ask me to drive her back to the airport. He let us pass through the police tape but asked us to spend the night inside. He didn't need to ask us twice. I can't imagine Diane slept much that night.

We showed up at my clinic the next morning. Diane had carried seven babies by then, twice as a surrogate, and she was very much at ease with the whole process. I had done my egg retrieval three days earlier and we had good embryos to transfer. The doctor did the transfer and then Diane and I spent the day together at my house. I made her lunch and learned about her kids and her life. She was divorced but on good terms with her ex-husband who was still an important part of her life.

She had five of her own children. She is one of eight siblings. Her mother, who I later met, was the biggest Packers fan I will likely ever meet. I thought that in a different context, Diane and I would just be friends. I dropped her back at the airport that evening. Two weeks later she was disappointed to learn that she was not pregnant. She seemed let down by her own body and she was clearly determined to make this happen the next time. I took the news in stride. I only knew failure, so it was just one more to process.

We agreed to try again in a few months. Diane travelled to Toronto. This time we arranged for her to stay in a hotel after the transfer to have a day to rest before heading home. She was convinced that the first time had failed because she had flown home that evening. David drove her to the airport the next day. It was the Sunday of the Masters golf tournament. At the airport she told him that she had a good feeling about this one and that she felt pregnant. All he could think was, "Please don't jinx this."

She did a home pregnancy test very early a week later. She called to let me know that she had been driving around Green Bay that afternoon consulting people on whether they thought the faint line on the pee stick indicated a pregnancy. She was confident that she was pregnant. She was very open at work and in her community that she was a surrogate. People seemed to be more than simply curious. They seemed to respect her for it. I felt lucky to be doing this with her. When we got the official blood test results from her doctor a week later, she was, indeed, very pregnant.

It was the end of April. Both Diane and Debbie were pregnant. We were expecting two children, a month apart, in December and the following January.

This all felt too good to be real. I am sure I had some element of post-traumatic stress disorder. David and I had been at this for so long and fertility treatments had become a routine part of our daily life. I was thirty-seven. I had done close to twenty medical procedures by then, injected myself with hundreds of needles, and had blood drawn from my veins so many times that I had tiny track marks in my arms.

I was practically a celebrity at my clinic. Other than the FBI and my federal tax bureau, there is no other place I would have wanted to become a household name less than my fertility clinic. They were nothing but good to me but by the time I was done with treatments, I never wanted to step foot in that place again.

We had kept the fact that we were trying with two surrogates to ourselves and our doctors. Managing anyone's feelings and expectations beyond our own was not something that we had the energy for. We planned to tell our surrogates more details about each other once they each cleared the first trimester.

With no medical appointments on the horizon, we arranged a week away. We spent a few days in the U.S. sailing with two close friends, David and Chisholm, who had uprooted their lives a couple of years earlier to sail around the world and had now settled in New York. We spent the second half of the week at a cottage with Mary and Timon. We ate, we laughed, the men drove race cars for the first time at a track near where we were staying. We left our troubles at home that weekend. But trouble tracked us down.

Shortly before we packed up to head home my cell phone rang. Diane was on the other end in tears. It was hard to understand her but eventually I understood that she had lost the baby. She had started to bleed that morning and had gone to the hospital. They did an ultrasound and there was no sign or sound of the baby. She was nine weeks along. They told her that she had miscarried.

I was used to processing disappointment, but this felt different. I felt foolish for having let my guard down. I should have known that something difficult was around the corner.

We packed off our friends and then sat together before getting ready to leave. Debbie was nearing the end of the first trimester, which in and of itself was a big milestone, but being on the other side of infertility still seemed like a long way off. It felt so sad.

As Debbie cleared the first trimester, we began making arrangements for her obstetrical care and delivery. If I had learned anything from working with a smaller regional hospital with my first surrogate, it is that not all hospitals are created equal. I wanted Debbie to be delivering at an urban hospital with experience around surrogacy. My fertility specialist had very kindly arranged for the pregnancy to be supervised by a well-respected obstetrician at a hospital near my home in Toronto. He let me know at the outset that, as a favour to my specialist, he had agreed to jointly manage Debbie's care with her local hospital. This was an unusual arrangement that few doctors would agree to because of the risks and liability involved in managing a pregnancy with another doctor. I guessed that my fertility doctor had compromising pictures on the other guy.

In truth, the other guy was an excellent physician and I felt lucky and appreciative. Debbie and I had agreed that doctors' appointments would be at her local hospital but, closer to her due date, she would travel to Toronto for appointments and for the delivery.

Debbie provided regular email updates on how the pregnancy was progressing and small details on how the baby was doing that made David and I feel part of the experience. As spring gave way to summer, we started getting used to the idea of becoming parents again. I was surprised at how normal it felt. I was able to treat this pregnancy like a typical pregnancy, processing the standard risks and information that come along with that. I did not feel neurotic.

If anything, I worried that I was too detached. I wondered if having another child, and a daughter at that, felt like a betrayal of Sam. How do you move forward from the death of one child to celebrate the arrival of another? How do you raise a daughter in the shadow of her sister who won't get to do any of the things she will be able to do? Every time she hit a milestone, would I be thinking of Sam? I kept these thoughts to myself as David and I began to prepare for the December arrival of another child.

All of Sam's baby stuff was gone. We didn't try to get it back. It just felt too painful. We were starting over.

CHAPTER SIX

The Great Vanishing Act

I WAS WORKING IN MY OFFICE one afternoon, about two and a half months after Diane's miscarriage, when the phone rang. Diane was calling from her doctor's office. She was practically screaming. I thought she might be hurt. I heard the words "miracle" and "baby".

Eventually I understood that she was telling me that she was still pregnant, that she had never miscarried. She may have been carrying twins and had miscarried one. Diane had gone back several times to the hospital to let them know that she still felt pregnant. Each time they told her she was likely experiencing a "fantasy pregnancy" where her mind can't accept the miscarriage and her body mimics the symptoms and they sent her home.

I got on the phone with the doctor who told me that they had finally done an ultrasound, nine weeks after the miscarriage diagnosis, and discovered that Diane was, in fact, eighteen weeks pregnant. She was carrying a baby girl.

I reflected on the use of the word "miracle." It was only a miracle if the baby had actually disappeared and then reappeared. She had been there all along. She was just waiting for someone to notice.

I don't remember much from that afternoon, but I do remember how I felt. It was like winning the lottery. You can fantasize about something like this happening but deep down you know it's just a dream. And yet someone out there does win.

This time it was us.

This was joyful news but there was a practical dimension that was tricky. In Canada, our surrogate pregnancies were covered by public health insurance. There was no cost to us for any of the medical care for Debbie's pregnancy.

We needed private health insurance for the U.S. There was a standard insurance plan for surrogacy that could be purchased, but it had to be in place by the end of the first trimester. It was expensive, approximately US$10,000, but it covered many of the pregnancy costs and provided additional coverage if something went wrong. You could get a policy in the second trimester but the longer you waited, the more it cost. It was also conditional on acceptance by the insurance company. We planned to purchase insurance for Diane in the first trimester but when she miscarried, we didn't follow through with that plan.

Unfortunately, by the time we learned that she was still pregnant, between Diane's age and the advanced stage of the pregnancy, no one would insure her. This left us financially vulnerable. David and I would be on the hook for hundreds of thousands of dollars in medical costs if something went wrong.

I flew to Green Bay that weekend for the belated pre-natal testing. In the ultrasound, the baby looked perfectly normal. Diane and I joked that, under the circumstances, it was fortuitous that I ended up with a surrogate who lived like a nun. Diane doesn't smoke or drink and, between working and raising two young children, she had no time to date.

By then, Debbie, back in Canada, was twenty-two weeks pregnant and it was time to talk to Diane and Debbie about each other.

Telling Diane did not feel like a big deal. She had confirmed in one of our early conversations that she would be fine if David and I did this with two surrogates. We were having a cup of tea in her kitchen, playing with her two dogs, when I broached the subject. I told her that David and I were incredibly happy about her pregnancy and that we were also expecting a second baby around the same time.

Diane was stunned. She seemed confused and hurt. I was equally confused by her reaction. She wanted to know why she was only finding out then. I explained that we had planned to tell both surrogates after the first trimester but when she miscarried there was no news to share. She wanted to know what her pregnancy meant to us if we were also expecting another child. I said that we could not be happier.

It did not matter what I said or how I tried to explain. She never raised her voice, never cried, or said an unkind word. But it was clear to me that she was deeply hurt and angry.

I understood that this was not a conversation that would get closure from establishing who was right and who was wrong. I couldn't walk in her shoes to understand why this mattered so much to her. She couldn't walk in mine. But I had decided at the outset of surrogacy that I did not want conflict to be an option in these relationships. David and I had deliberately chosen experienced surrogates who were strong women knowing that we would have to work through any issues that might arise together. It was important to me that I did not leave Green Bay with a fundamental breach in my relationship with Diane. I didn't worry about the baby. Diane would always do right by the baby. But Diane had lost trust in me.

I took her family out for dinner that night to an all-you-can-eat buffet. We laughed and joked throughout the meal. Diane kept pointing to vegetables on her plate, showing off her pregnancy diet. I enjoyed getting to know her family a bit and to see Diane in her own environment. But it didn't resolve the disconnect between us.

When I got on the plane the next day I was shattered. I had not expected Diane's reaction. I always wanted us to be able to look each other in the eyes with respect. I worried that we wouldn't be able to work through our differences.

Ultimately, we did, which was an enormous relief to me.

I wasn't in Green Bay for Diane's medical appointments but, like Debbie, she shared information and details that made David and I feel very connected to the pregnancy. She suggested that I might want to record songs of me singing that she could play to the baby so that she would recognize my voice. I told her that unless the baby had the option of ear plugs it was probably not a good idea.

CHAPTER SEVEN

The Fighter

I SAT ON OUR BACK DECK one day in early September reading and was startled to feel the breeze on my face. It washed over me like warm water and I realized that I hadn't felt a breeze, or much of anything, for that matter, since the night we left the hospital after saying goodbye to Sam. That was two years earlier. I was finally rejoining the land of the living.

The following weekend I went for a long run on a beautiful September Sunday. We had friends over for lunch. The sun streamed into our house from the street and it felt spectacular to be doing normal people things. Part way through lunch the phone rang. It was Debbie calling from her local hospital. She wanted me to speak with the doctor. The doctor explained that Debbie had come in that morning with some leaking fluid. She felt that it was likely just incontinence but to be prudent she wanted Debbie transported to Toronto to be at a hospital that was better equipped to manage a premature delivery in the off chance that it was anything problematic. Debbie was exactly twenty-eight weeks pregnant. I knew this was not good.

She was transported by air ambulance to Toronto and then transferred by land ambulance to Sunnybrook and Women's College

Hospital where we met her. She was calm, as she always was, but clearly discombobulated by the turn of events. We met with a team of doctors, who had taken a sample of the fluid to be tested, so that we could discuss the potential risks of a premature birth at this stage.

The doctors felt fairly confident, given what they had seen on the ultrasound, including a healthy, active baby and fetal sac full of liquid, that this was going to be urine and not amniotic fluid. They would not know for sure until they got the test results back in the morning. They explained that in a situation where it was a rupture of the fetal sac, a woman had a fifty-percent chance of going into labour within forty-eight hours. Because of this, they would administer a steroid shot to help speed up the baby's lung development. They explained to all of us the risks to the baby of being born this early. I listened intently to the doctor describe the risks of the baby dying in labour or shortly after birth, as well as the potential health impacts if she lived, including blindness, cerebral palsy, and brain damage. It was sobering, but I left the hospital that night with a sense that we would look back on that day as a bad scare. I expected Debbie would be released the next day and we would get back to our lives.

I couldn't have been more wrong. We met with the doctors the following morning. They confirmed that it was amniotic fluid. Debbie's fetal sac had ripped, and we needed to prepare for an imminent birth. Debbie was instructed to be on bed rest in the hospital until the baby came. If labour didn't happen in the next twenty-four hours, there was no way of predicting when it would. The doctors explained that eventually Debbie would get an infection, which would trigger labour in order to get the baby out of a place that was no longer safe for her to grow. It could be a day; it could be two months. They impressed upon us that at this stage every additional day in utero was critical for the baby's development.

Debbie did not complain but my heart ached for her. I came to the hospital each day with food, magazines, and other forms of entertainment but none of that could compensate for being away from her kids and her family. I came down the hospital hallway one evening and could hear her in the room quietly crying and speaking on the phone with a family member, telling them how scared and homesick she was. I knocked and she pulled herself together as if she had not been crying. When I asked her if there was anything that I could do to make this easier for her she said that she was fine but that she missed hearing the chirping of the two budgies she kept in her kitchen. This felt like code for "I just want to get back to my life." We both knew that the sooner that happened, the worse it was for the baby and the longer it was, the harder it was for her. I knew that she was doing everything she could do to bring the baby to term.

I left the hospital each night with the understanding that the hospital would call me if there were any important developments. Given what was at stake, waiting for my cell phone to ring was frightening. I had asked everyone not to call my phone. As luck would have it, that week I ended up with my first crank caller. An elderly gentleman called my number at random times day and night, telling me that I had stolen his telephone number. I had had the number for five years, so I knew that wasn't the case. Each time the phone rang my heart stopped. I pleaded with him to stop calling me. The phone went silent for a few days.

Debbie reached the twenty-nine-week mark on the Sunday after she was admitted. The aim was to get to thirty-two weeks, which would put the baby in a much lower risk category. We met with the doctors that morning to go through the risks once again. Debbie had a headache when I left the hospital that night and I went to bed with a bad feeling. The call came at five the next morning. I hoped it was my crank caller but a nurse on the other end told us it was time to come to the hospital. Debbie had gone into labour. David and I got dressed in silence. Neither of us could speak. As we stood in our garage in the dark, ready to get into our car, he hugged me. The only other person who knew how bad this felt was him.

We found Debbie in a small side room near the delivery rooms when we got to the hospital. She was fully in labour but had not been given an epidural, so she was in a lot of discomfort. Our original birth plan had been for Debbie's sister or mother to be her support person for the labour and for me to be in the delivery room. They clearly weren't going to make it. I had never been near a birth, so I didn't know how to be supportive. I spoke to a nurse to find out what I could do. Debbie was vomiting. The nurse told me to feed her ice chips, keep her hydrated and squeeze her hips together when she had contractions to help manage the pain.

I couldn't generate enough strength with my arms, so I spent the next couple of hours straddling her with my legs and feeding her ice chips. I did not want her to go through this. I did not want to be going through this. There is often a closeness in surrogacy, given the unique nature of the relationship, that transcends the limited extent that you actually know each other. But I had never met her husband or her children. I didn't know what food or music she liked or what her favourite colour was. That morning I knew that we were effectively two strangers going through this intimate, vulnerable, frightening experience together.

I went into the hallway at one point to collect my thoughts. The conversation with the doctors the night before, explaining the risks to the baby, ran on a loop in my head. When I stripped it all down and thought about what I wanted for my child, it was simple. She didn't need to fly to the moon or run a marathon. I just wanted her to be able to develop meaningful relationships and kick a soccer ball. To make friends and to run around. If nothing else, for her sake, I wanted that. I would have cashed in all my chips for just those two things.

Our obstetrician was not on shift that day, but he came to check on us. He found me standing outside Debbie's room with tears running down my face. He asked me what was wrong. If I had feared earlier in the pregnancy that I was too detached, now I felt like I was in the fight of my life. I wanted this baby more than anything in the world.

I told him that I couldn't go through this again. I didn't think David or I could survive another loss. He put his hands on my shoulders, looked me straight in the eye and said the five most comforting words anyone has ever said to me. "She's going to be fine." I don't know if he had any medical basis to say that. I didn't care. He said it with complete confidence. It got me through that day.

* * *

After six hours of labour, Debbie was transferred into a special delivery room attached to the Level III Neo-Natal Intensive Care Unit (NICU), where they transferred the most critical care babies after birth. We started to follow her. Someone told us that we could not be there. The doctors would come talk to us after the delivery. Confused and scared as Debbie was wheeled away, we went to see the head nurse to ask where we could wait. She asked us why we were not in the delivery room. We told her someone had told us we couldn't be in the room and she said to put on some scrubs and to get in there.

When we got into the delivery room, a nurse was on the phone saying in a loud and urgent voice to the doctor, "It is happening, you need to get here now." Minutes later, the baby came flying out like a rocket. Someone caught her like a football in what seemed to be mid-air, put her on a table and wheeled her out of the room. We didn't know what happened next. I assumed that it would be hours and maybe days before we could see her. I had no idea where she went or what they would do with her. I didn't know if she was on the verge of death or doing fine. A nurse popped her head in just then and said, "Do you want to meet your daughter?" She beckoned us to a side room where I laid eyes on the tiniest human I had ever seen. She weighed less than three pounds. She was a bag of bones, wrinkly all over. I will give her this: she was extremely flexible. You could twist her limbs into a pretzel.

I felt panicky watching her struggle to breathe. I asked the nurse to help her. She told me she was waiting to see if she could breathe without assistance. They had expected her to be intubated and breathe with a ventilator machine. Suddenly her torso heaved, she took in a deep breath and her chest started to move up and down as she inhaled and exhaled. She had figured it out on her own.

One hurdle down. Another hundred to go.

I had no experience to know how to read her progress but I was picking up signs that she was doing surprisingly well. The staff were laughing at how crabby she was as they tried unsuccessfully to get a tiny IV into her miniscule veins. They took pictures of her in the first moments of her life. All of these things gave me comfort that, as far as a kid at twenty-nine weeks was going to be, she was fine, so far. She was and is a fighter. We named her Georgia, a name we both loved and the same name as Chella's daughter, my goddaughter, who we also love.

I checked on Debbie. She was okay but exhausted. We were all exhausted.

David and I met with a doctor who explained more about next steps and what would happen from here. I felt sick to my stomach, but I knew that this would be a marathon and not a sprint. We would have to learn to live with a lot of unknowns and take it day to day. They expected that Georgia had contracted an infection in the birth canal, which was the most immediate threat to her survival. She was covered in bacteria when she came out. They took a sample and said they would not know until they got the full lab results in a week. In the meantime, they had started her on a general antibiotic and would tailor it once they had better information on what the infection might be. We were as surprised as the doctors when the lab results came in a week later and showed that there was no infection. Lady Luck was finally making an appearance. They had done a brain scan to check for hemorrhaging or lesions and it looked like she had none. They would do another in a week.

The doctor told us that, as the birth mother, Debbie would have all decision-making authority for Georgia. I almost fell off my chair. I explained to him that she was not the mother and would not want that responsibility. If anyone was making life or death decisions for our child, it was me and David. He said that he had never encountered a situation like this and that he would seek legal advice from the hospital.

I was appalled by the suggestion, but I knew he was navigating as best he could. We told him that there was no disputing that David was the birth father and he would make the decisions if necessary. The doctor went to see Debbie. He confirmed that she did not want decision-making responsibility and had verbally consented to relinquish her authority. He also let us know that they wanted to start Georgia on a feeding tube, a tiny wire run through her nose down into her tummy, and that the best possible food for her was breast milk. They were in the process of trying to create a breast milk bank at the hospital, where mothers could donate breast milk for other babies. But they hadn't set it up yet. The biggest risk for all of the babies in the NICU in the first few weeks is infection, particularly in their intestinal tissue. The risk was greatly reduced with breast milk. He impressed upon us the seriousness of the situation.

Debbie and I had discussed the possibility of pumping breast milk as part of our contract negotiations. She did not want to pump, and I was fine with that at the time. This was obviously very different. I knew how scared and drained she was. This experience had pushed her far out of her comfort zone and she just wanted to go home. I went to see her and conveyed what the doctor had said. Her answer had potentially life-altering consequences for my child but, like so many of the experiences on this journey, I had no control over how things played out. There was nothing we could do if she said no. She seemed surprised by the request. She looked at me with eyes that said, "Please don't ask me to do this." And then, after what felt like minutes but was probably no more than a few seconds, she said yes. The nurses came in immediately to get her started pumping so that Georgia could be fed.

Two days later, Debbie was discharged from the hospital with a pumping machine to take home. She didn't get to reclaim her body, her life, her sleep, or her independence as most surrogates do after giving birth. She pumped seven times a day for four months. She organized a system to put the milk in freezer bags and bought coolers to transport it once a week to Toronto. David or one of our friends or family members would meet her or one of her family members in a parking lot at night half-way between our homes. We used to laugh that people must be placing bets on what was stashed in the coolers that were shuttled back and forth by our sixty-five-year-old mothers—drugs or casseroles.

We would bring the milk to the NICU for the nurses to prepare feedings for Georgia. After two months I broached the topic of stopping with Debbie. By then she was a pumping machine. She had produced enough milk to get Georgia well past her actual due date and Georgia was doing well. Characteristic of the humanity she showed throughout the whole process, Debbie wanted to continue. Georgia was not her child. None of this had unfolded in a way that was comfortable for her, but Georgia's best interests were always her focus. She is one of the main reasons why Georgia is who she is today. David and I would take a bullet for that woman.

We camped out beside Georgia's incubator in the NICU. An older, very experienced nurse was caring for her. When Georgia was only two days old, the nurse asked me if I had held her yet. I looked at her like she was high. I told her that I had not. Given a choice, I would have opted not to hold her for a while longer. She just seemed too fragile. The nurse didn't give me a choice. She told me to remove my top so Georgia could lie on my skin. I made a mental note to buy better bras going forward.

She helped me remove her from her incubator and, as if reading my mind, she said, "Don't worry, you're not going to drop her." She placed her on my chest. Her little heart was racing. I thought she was going to have a heart attack. And then, just as the nurse had said, her heart slowed down to a more regular rhythm and she nuzzled into me like we had known each other forever. She couldn't be out of her incubator for long, but I will always remember that feeling of skin to skin contact with her tiny body. It felt like the most gentle and intimate experience I had ever had with another person. We have a picture of David holding her in those first few days when she wrapped her tiny hand around his pinky finger. It looks like she is holding the finger of a giant.

A few dozen babies were jammed in to the cramped NICU with a little space around each incubator for medical equipment and a chair for someone to sit in. It looked terrible but somehow it worked. The hospital was on the cusp of moving to a new location with state of the art NICU facilities, but that was months away. There was no defined space around each incubator, so you created your own little world around your baby. You were mindful of other people and what they were going through. We talked in low voices to give each other privacy but you could overhear conversations. Many of the babies were even younger and smaller than Georgia. It was clear that some of them would not make it. We could hear parents talking quietly to their babies, saying goodbye, in a room full of people during the most heart-breaking moments of their lives. I imagine many of them felt like I did with Sam and just wanted to get down on their knees and plead for a different outcome. Please take me and not my child. I will do anything you ask of me. Just tell me what you want. The most powerless feeling in the world may be knowing there is nothing you can do to save your child.

Six months earlier the NICU had been temporarily shut down following an infectious illness outbreak. We always wore hospital gowns and slippers and disinfected our hands and arms in an anteroom before we entered the NICU. If you were sick, they implored you to stay away for fear of spreading germs. I got a cold at one point and I had to spend those few days watching Georgia through a window. It felt like she was a million miles away.

Georgia had a soft layer of hair covering her body. She looked like a tiny rubber chicken but felt more like a baby duckling. Her eyes weren't locked into their sockets and her eyeballs rolled around. She couldn't swallow so she was still fed through a tube. She sometimes didn't remember to breathe and was hooked up to wires and machines that sounded alarms for nurses to tap her on the back and remind her. She couldn't regulate her temperature, so she grew in a temperature-controlled incubator. The risks to her survival were many.

We were stressed and scared but the medical staff had given us every reason to be hopeful. Each night we left the hospital with the understanding that if there were any significant developments overnight the hospital would contact us.

For the many weeks that Georgia was in the hospital, David typically arrived around 5:30 every morning to hang out with her for a few hours before he went to work. On the fifth morning he showed up and she was gone. There was an empty spot where her incubator had been. A nurse across the room, seeing his anguished face and realizing that he thought she had died in the night, rushed over to tell him that she had been moved upstairs to the Level II NICU room, which was for babies who were stable and doing well. They had to admit a new baby overnight and were short of beds. Out of all of the babies in the Level III NICU, Georgia was doing well enough to be moved. When David called to let me know, I could not have felt prouder if he had told me that our child had just run a four-minute mile.

We settled in to a new normal with Georgia's birth. We began to act like new parents.

When David posted the first pictures of Georgia on Facebook, our former surrogate Michelle connected with him to inquire about her. She also had a newborn. It became clear through their exchange that, following our unsuccessful attempts, she had her husband reverse his vasectomy so that she could have another child. As much as pregnancy seems unimaginable to many women struggling with infertility, for surrogates it is often the opposite. They expect to get pregnant. I wondered if it was important for Michelle to prove to herself that she was not the cause of our "failure."

After five weeks at the first critical care hospital where Georgia was delivered, she was strong enough to be moved to a different hospital, St. Michael's Hospital, as soon as a NICU bed was available. This was a big step because it meant she needed less care. We had been told that we would be given advanced warning. For me, advanced warning meant a day or two. Instead, I got a call at work one afternoon from a nurse telling me that a bed had freed up and they were moving Georgia within the hour. I grabbed my bag and ran to the hospital. I worried that if I wasn't there, they might misplace her in transit like a piece of luggage. They were in the process of moving her incubator into the elevator when I got there and then they loaded her into an ambulance. I sat in the front for the drive. The hospital entrance, located in one of the grittiest parts of Toronto, was blocked so the ambulance parked on the street. They wheeled her incubator along a busy downtown street, weaving their way past streetcars, heavy traffic and curious onlookers. I thought I might faint.

Georgia was taken up the elevator to the NICU and a very skilled nurse took over. She was an Albanian doctor who had emigrated to Canada a decade earlier. She was unable to practice as a doctor in Canada, but she had re-qualified as a neonatal nurse. No sooner had she prepared her new incubator and placed the baby inside than Georgia had explosive diarrhea. She has always had impeccable timing. I worried that Georgia would end up on the wrong side of the staff. But the nurse was professional, patient, and kind. She cleaned Georgia and prepared the incubator once again.

I came to know this nurse well. As we learned more about each other's stories, I discovered that, shortly after she was born, she had been given by her parents to her Aunt and Uncle, who were infertile. When she discovered that I had already lost a child and that I had a sister who had twins, she asked me why I hadn't just asked Sharon to give me one of her children. I told her that would be unusual in my culture. I also thought it would be a potentially awkward conversation. She shrugged and said, "All you can do is ask." She had a point.

Over the next month the world fell away as we hunkered down with our daughter and the doctors and nurses taught us how to parent. She was still attached to wires and machines so alarms would go off all the time. The nurses would tell us to look at our child, not the machines. They encouraged us to learn her signs to meet her needs. They removed the feeding tube after six weeks and taught her how to feed, and us how to give her a bottle. They were preparing us for life as a family beyond the NICU.

I have never felt safer as a parent than in that place.

David, who is not a very chatty person unless you are talking about coffee, Dimpflmeier bread, or sports, knew everyone. Their stories. Their kids' names. He was there in the wee hours of the morning before work and late at night before bed. He knew every nurse from every shift. They loved him. He was basically the mayor of the NICU. He had started growing a mustache while Georgia was in the hospital. One day, a few of the nurses pulled me aside. They wanted to discreetly tell me that if David was growing a mustache to look more like a dad, they didn't think it was a good look for him. I explained that he was growing the mustache for an international prostate cancer fundraiser called "Movember." I told them we knew it made him look like a European porn star but that he would shave it at the end of November.

It was good to know they had his back.

This NICU was a communal place. It was full of people from different walks of life. We could tell that one of the babies was born to a girl living on the street. A social worker seemed to be working with her to move the baby into foster care. There was another young mother who looked to be in her teens. Her boyfriend showed up for the first time one day to meet his child. He bristled at the many NICU rules and regulations. He didn't want to be told how to behave or what to do. He argued with the staff and left angrily. The next time he came, I watched a nurse patiently and caringly work to make him feel comfortable and start to bond with his baby. He came more regularly after that. There was a couple from a very wealthy family who had had twins through IVF; they were born prematurely, a common risk with twins.

Our paths may never have crossed outside of that room but inside the NICU we shared a common bond. In that room every child received the same care, rich or poor, black or white, boy or girl, they were equals. But outside that room, David and I were conscious that their lives would take very different paths. The single most important factor influencing outcomes for preemies, aside from their gestational age at birth, is their parents' level of education. With two lawyer parents I knew that Georgia was starting from a very advantageous place. That may be the only time in her life when she would agree that having two lawyers for parents was a benefit.

Many of the babies were in the NICU only briefly. They might need to be monitored for a night or two because of low birth weights or after a difficult delivery. You could sometimes hear parents of these babies re-counting their labour and delivery stories in harrowing detail to family and friends. For many of them it probably was the worst experience of their lives. David and I used to look at each other. We thought of Sam. We thought of the parents we heard saying goodbye to their babies at the first NICU. We knew that none of this was like the movies. You don't always end up with a great dinner party story. It often doesn't turn out okay.

But for Georgia it did.

Ten weeks after she came into the world, we unhooked her from all of the wires and machines and monitors and wheeled her into a private room in the NICU for our last night. I was scared to put her in a car the next day, let alone bring her home and raise her without a SWAT team of medical professionals.

The vivid memories of my fear are only eclipsed by the even more vivid memories of sleeping on the least comfortable pull-out bed I hope to ever encounter. Well played, NICU.

I wandered around the unit all night wondering how on earth we were going to do this on our own.

CHAPTER EIGHT

Game Day

IN THAT LATE FALL OF 2008, as we prepared for Georgia's homecoming, we were also getting ready for the birth of her sister in Green Bay.

Diane was scheduled for a C-section in early January around her January 5 due date. I asked her to broach the subject of moving up the date with her doctor. She raised the issue, but the doctor refused. She clearly felt that I was trying to move the date so that it would not interfere with my Christmas holidays. I asked to speak with her directly. I explained that I was concerned that Diane, who usually went into labour before her due date and who had had unexpected complications late in one of her pregnancies, could go into spontaneous labour and be rushed to the hospital for an emergency C-section. I said that between Christmas and bad winter weather, I worried about staffing issues and wanted to avoid an unscheduled procedure. I explained that we had lost a child in labour delivery and that I knew that things did not always go as planned. I told her we had a baby born at twenty-nine weeks who had just come home from the NICU and that my sole focus was the safety of the baby. Once she understood, I could feel her tone soften. She scheduled the C-section for December 22.

Before then, there were important legal issues that needed to be navigated, given that we were doing this outside of Canada. For Georgia, we went to court after her birth to finalize the legal documentation. This could not be done in Ontario before her birth. In Wisconsin, you could apply for a pre-birth order, the legal document declaring us as the parents. This meant that right after the birth we could apply for a final order which, in turn, allowed us to apply for the formal birth certificate. These final steps could happen within the first hours after birth and we would need all of these documents to be able to bring the baby across the border.

In the weeks leading up to the birth, David and I worked with a U.S. lawyer to get the documents ready and to prepare for a court hearing by telephone. Obtaining the order was not just a formality. The judge, the lawyer, and Diane were present in the courtroom. The judge asked us questions over the phone around why we were doing this. He asked Diane questions to ensure she was doing this of her own free will and that she understood that she would be relinquishing all rights to the child once there was a pre-birth order in place. He was very professional, and the hearing was straightforward, but I was conscious of the enormous power that he held over all of our lives that day.

When my dad asked me about a month before the delivery date who I was bringing with me to Green Bay, he should not have been surprised when I told him that he was coming. Although, when he asked the question, I realized that I had made the decision a long time ago, even if I hadn't actually communicated it to him. Like a kid, I assumed my dad would be there if I needed him.

Georgia was just home from the hospital. David and I agreed that he would stay with Georgia in Toronto. My dad checked the date and told me that he was scheduled to be in Abu Dhabi for work. I explained to him why I needed him there. I didn't need him for moral support or for his sense of humour. It had been a long road getting here. Between the birth, the drive home, the legal issues bringing a newborn across the border, there was no end of things that could go wrong. I told him it was his job to get us home safely.

Growing up, my dad was our driver. He drove us to sleepovers and sports practices. He drove us to and from universities. He moved us into and out of dorm rooms and apartments. He used to say the pay was pretty bad, but the company made up for it. I'm not so sure about that.

This was going to be the most important drive of my life. He nodded and left the living room. Half an hour later he came back and let me know that he had cleared his schedule and was coming.

On December 21st, I kissed David and Georgia goodbye and drove the hour and a half to my parents' farm to meet my dad and begin the drive to Green Bay. We needed to stop in Chicago to pick up my sister Sam, who was flying in from Boston to join us. We took his car and I kept harping on him to make sure we had a full tank of gas before we left. A few months earlier, while sitting in a government meeting, I learned that the contract to refurbish the roadside service stations on Ontario's main highway—Highway 401, the same the one we were about to take—would put many of those service stations out of commission for renovations at exactly the same time that we'd be driving past them. It wouldn't be a great time to need gas. I remember one of my colleagues saying that our summer tourism campaign slogan should be: "Cross your legs Ontario, it's going to be a long drive".

He was right, it was a long drive. As we approached the border crossing in Detroit, I started to get nervous. I asked my dad how he wanted to answer questions around the purpose of our visit. I was so attuned to the misperceptions and judgments around surrogacy that I approached every interaction where I needed to explain things to a stranger with unease. He just said, "We keep it simple and tell the truth." When the customs official asked us the purpose of our visit, my dad said we were coming for the birth of his granddaughter. He asked us where she was being born. My dad said Green Bay. The official said, "Please don't name her Cheesehead," a nickname for Packers fans. We told him that was good advice. We rolled up our window and we were back on the road. Honestly, I don't know how my dad does it.

We made a quick stop in Chicago to collect my sister and arrived in Green Bay late that evening to check into our hotel. We were all staying together in a room with a little kitchenette. Most stores and restaurants were closed by the time we arrived, and the hotel only had vending machines. We went out to find some groceries and had a simple dinner in our room.

I was picking up Diane at six the following morning to bring her to the hospital. Between my dad's snoring, my sister storming up and down the hallway in the middle of the night trying to locate ear plugs, and my worrying about the delivery the next day, I did not sleep.

I had never experienced a normal birth. Our first child died in labour. Our second child came eleven weeks early and lived in an incubator for the first two months of her life. Our third child, this one, disappeared for a considerable stretch of the pregnancy. I wasn't consumed with what could go wrong, but as I went to bed that night, I recognized that it isn't over until it's over.

I picked Diane up at home. It was a bitterly cold morning and the sky was very dark and piercingly clear, like black glass. Diane, as expected, was calm and confident. Pregnancy was a joyful experience for her. She only knew success. When we arrived at the hospital entrance there was not a car in sight, but a valet asked for my keys to bring my car to the parking lot about thirty feet on the other side of the road. I told him that I could park it myself. He looked at me like I had two heads. Valet parking was part of the hospital package.

As David and I had discovered, a pregnancy in the U.S. is a very expensive endeavour. At one point, I spoke with the obstetrician who had managed Georgia's delivery about the possibility of Diane delivering in Canada. He advised against it because we would be paying out of pocket for the delivery and he felt it would be too expensive. I asked him how much it would cost. He said around $10,000 (Can.) for a C-section. I told him that in the U.S. we were going to pay well over $25,000 (U.S.).

I helped Diane get settled into an enormous room that looked like a luxury hotel suite. It had a giant flat screen TV. You could have hosted a cocktail party in there. I thought of the cramped NICU where Georgia was transferred after she was born, which looked like a bomb shelter, notwithstanding the good care she received. I thought of how different the two countries are. In the U.S., this was a business . . . and Diane and I were paying customers.

My dad and sister arrived at the hospital. Diane's mom and youngest daughter arrived. We all waited together in Diane's hospital room. It is hard to do justice to Diane's mother. As you would expect of the matriarch of a family of eight children, she was a pistol. Sharp, funny, strong, and tough. She was also dressed in full Green Bay Packers gear from head to toe. I had seen ardent sports fans with wigs and jerseys and face paint and other paraphernalia at games. I had never seen anything like this. She was wearing a Packers parka, turtleneck sweater, cardigan, earrings, gold chain, green slacks and Packers winter boots. I cannot speak for her undergarments, but she was as visibly associated with the home team as any fan I have ever seen. And this was not game day. It was just a regular Monday for Diane's mom.

I was very wired that morning. In addition to the birth I was also dealing with a difficult work issue that hit very close to home. A small group of senior government officials had made a series of awful decisions that had derailed the adoption of a child by an

Ontario couple. I had been fighting internally to have the situation brought to an appropriate resolution. I wanted the couple to be treated fairly. On the precipice of being forced to abandon the adoption because they were unable to get the relevant documents in time to travel to meet their baby, the couple took the government to court for an emergency family court hearing. The judges provided an immediate ruling directing the government to urgently do what these officials had been refusing to do for weeks. They were justifiably scathing about the government's handling of the matter. A week out from the court decision, the government still hadn't complied with the court order.

That morning the government was being brought back to court on a contempt of court motion. I had never seen anything like this in government. It was a terrible situation and I was going back and forth on email and on the phone with colleagues to try to resolve it. I hate unfairness generally, and this situation was profoundly unfair for the couple involved. It felt ironic that such an unjust professional issue was thrust into such a fundamental day in my personal life. I tried to do justice to each experience. Shortly before the scheduled court appearance, the court finally received the appropriate assurances that the court order was being complied with and the couple would receive the relevant papers to be able to travel to China for the adoption. The contempt motion was dropped.

I feel angry to this day for what that couple had to go through. But I knew that morning that they were about to embark on the best journey of their life—becoming parents. I reflected on our respective situations and how little control you sometimes have over that journey when so much of it is in the hands of others.

The C-section, originally scheduled for 9 a.m., had to be moved a few times that morning for emergency C-sections. I was slightly nervous because we had a long drive back to Canada the next day and the later we left Green Bay, the later we reached home. They prepared Diane for the procedure and wheeled her into the delivery room at noon. She wasn't simply calm. She was downright excited.

She had very kindly arranged for me and another person of my choosing to be with her for the delivery. Her mom might have liked to be there, but they wanted us to have this experience. I had asked my dad a few weeks earlier if he wanted to be in the delivery room. He said that he would. I couldn't tell whether he was saying it to be supportive or whether he genuinely wanted to be there. When my mom delivered my sisters and I in the late sixties and seventies, having a dad in the delivery room was about as common as having a Mariachi band. I thought that maybe he was curious.

I got dressed in scrubs. I let my dad know that if he wanted to come in for the birth then he needed to get scrubbed up. He suggested that I let my sister go instead.

I settled onto a stool beside Diane. There was a sheet covering most of her body so I could only see her head. My sister came into the room to join us. Diane beckoned her over and before I could say anything, she popped a videorecorder into her hand and asked her to record the surgery. I am sure my sister wanted to say no—she must have thought that I had planned it—but she dutifully took the device and positioned herself in the corner of the room. I looked at her a few times during the procedure and saw that her hands were shaking. All I could think was that I had dodged a bullet. That could have been my father.

I listened as the doctors and nurses bantered throughout the operation. They were relaxed so I was relaxed. When they finally pulled the baby out, Diane directed the nurses to bring her to me. A nurse placed her in my arms. I was struck by how much she looked like her sister, Sam.

In one of the great birth announcements of all time, my dad sent an email to share the news of a safe delivery to my mom and my sisters. He *copied* David, who has never let him live that down.

It was a Roman Catholic hospital. I wondered if we would run into any difficulties with the staff given that this was a surrogacy. At one point, a nun came in to check on Diane. The room was packed with people, including Diane's family, me, my dad, my sister, and the baby, laughing like it was a party. The nun wanted to know if the mother needed anything and she approached Diane. Diane directed her to me, holding the baby in my arms, trying to give her a bottle. Diane said she was just the carrier and I was the mother. We joked later on that the nun probably thought we were all going straight to hell. In reality, she was a bit confused but totally professional. There was one nurse, however, who was openly hostile. She was curt in her answers to my questions and could hardly look at me. I don't know what her issues were. I imagine she disagreed with what we were doing. I didn't let her take up too much of my mental space but her disdain for me was obvious. Sam agreed. Ironically, we realized much later on that we had inadvertently captured her scowling at me in one of the photos in the recovery room.

Within minutes of the birth I was asked to provide a name for the baby so that the lawyer could file a final birth order application and get us the birth certificate. I had imagined I would have some time with the baby first. That wasn't going to be possible. She was six minutes old and she needed a name.

One name was already a contender.

During the delivery, Diane's mom, daughter, and my father had waited together in the hallway. It turns out that leaving Diane's mother and my father unchaperoned was a mistake.

Diane's mom had vigorously campaigned in the hallway for the name Bretta after the famous Green Bay quarterback Brett Favre. Admittedly, he is an excellent quarterback and I have been a Green

Bay Packers' fan my whole life. I am pretty sure I got connected to the Packers through the show *Happy Days*. It was set in Milwaukee. Green Bay was their team. If the Packers were good enough for Fonzie, they were good enough for me.

By the time I emerged from the delivery room with the baby, this thing had legs. Nurses were already calling her Bretta. They had practically drawn up the birth certificate. My dad, who was the person tasked with delivering the paperwork to the courthouse, seemed way too comfortable with the idea.

But that was not this baby's destiny. David and I had discussed a few names. He had given me carte blanche to make a game-time decision. When I looked at the baby, she looked like a Sadie. I used to joke that when you heard the name Sadie, you were either talking about a ninety-year-old or a kid under the age of ten. The name went out of fashion for eighty years, but it was making a comeback.

And Sadie it was.

We settled into Diane's recovery room for the next twenty-four hours. Sadie had to spend the night in the hospital nursery. My biggest fear when they wheeled her out of the recovery room was that they would accidentally switch her and another baby, even though the babies had hospital bracelets. I kept asking the nurses how they could be so sure that would not happen. When I laid eyes on the only two babies in the nursery, one pale and bald as a cue ball and the other with olive skin and a full head of jet-black hair, I understood why the nurses thought I was hilarious. I spent the night shuttling back and forth between the nursery and Diane's room.

We received the final birth certificate the morning of December 23. All we needed was the discharge from the hospital so that we could start the drive home. At exactly the twenty-four-hour mark following the birth, they discharged Sadie. We said our goodbyes. Diane's mom gave Sadie a beautiful baby blanket that she had knitted for her. It is one of our family's most treasured possessions.

I felt lucky to have met her and so respectful that she had raised a daughter like Diane. Diane asked to hold Sadie one last time. I loved how much she cared for her and also how consciously she defined her boundaries. This birth meant something special to her. She was, and still is, curious and caring about Sadie. But she has her own kids. She knows what it feels like to be a parent and to love your kid that way. This was not that.

CHAPTER NINE

The Kindness of Strangers

THE FOUR OF US PILED INTO my dad's car. We knew a
storm was coming and that we had a window of opportunity
to leave Green Bay, after which we could be snowed in for up
to a week. I did not want to discover how, if we got stuck there, we
would manage a newborn in a hotel room for a week. We couldn't
travel by plane until Sadie was a week old, so I had stockpiled for-
mula and diapers for the ten-hour drive back to my parents' farm to
join my mom, David, Georgia, and my sisters.

It was clear skies when we left the hospital, but the snow hit
earlier than we expected and with greater intensity. Between Green
Bay, Milwaukee, and Chicago, much of the drive is on the western
edge of Lake Michigan. The driving conditions down that particular
stretch were terrible. There were snow squalls and cars in the ditch.
For a time, the other side of the highway, which was directly on the
lake side, was closed off. We drove slowly, stopping only so I could
unstrap Sadie from her car seat and feed her a bottle every few hours.
I tried one feeding without stopping and she projectile vomited onto
the passenger seat. My dad was quiet and very focused on the road.

There was no one I would have felt safer driving with than him. Other than being a very good driver, I knew he had a lot at stake with two of his daughters and his new granddaughter in the car.

We had been driving for about twelve hours, inching along at about twenty-five miles an hour when, just outside Michigan City, Indiana, we got a flat tire. The snowstorm was getting worse and stopping now meant that we would have to find somewhere to stay to wait out the storm for at least the next few days. My heart sank. We travelled a few miles on the flat, looking for a motel. I was trying not to cry thinking about me, my dad and my sister holed up in a motel far from home taking care of Sadie. We ended up at a ramp that led down to a gas station. My dad navigated the car to the station. He wanted to change the tire, but he couldn't find the spare in the trunk. He went inside the gas station store to see if anyone could help him. It was around midnight, cold and windy with freezing rain and half a foot of slush on the ground. He emerged a few minutes later with a young man, a former U.S. Marine, who worked as a clerk in the store. He started to poke around the back of the car, looking for the spare. They got out the manual and realized that the spare was in a special compartment under the floor with access from deep inside the car.

My dad and the man began to unpack the car to access the tire. They needed to stash the luggage in the front of the car while they changed the tire so that our belongings wouldn't get soaked outside. The man was startled to find me and a newborn in the back seat. He apologized for disturbing us and took care to move everything carefully so that we wouldn't get hurt. He tried to keep the doors shut as much as possible so we wouldn't be cold.

They worked together under difficult conditions for over an hour. The man insisted that he, not my sixty-six-year-old father, get under the car to make the actual tire change. When they finished, they were both soaked, their fingers were frozen, and they were shivering with cold. I collected all of the cash we had in the car, about $100, so my dad could give it to him. I could hear the two of them going back and forth outside. I thought there must be a disagreement over money. I wanted to kick myself for not having thought of setting a price at the outset. It was a horrible job and I would have happily paid him more, but we only had the cash that we had.

I will never forget what happened next. My dad got back in the car. He said the man would not accept any payment. My dad insisted that he take the money to buy a Christmas present for his family. He said he didn't have a wife and his parents were dead. He said he could tell that this was an important drive for us, and he was happy to be of help. My dad told him that he was our Christmas miracle. He asked if there was anything at all that he could do for him. The man said that if my dad wanted to do something, he could write to his boss and tell him that he had done a good job. My dad was more than happy to do that when he got back to Canada.

It was a small but powerful act of kindness that I carry with me to this day. You can find heroes in unexpected places. He was our hero that night.

We continued the drive throughout the night, crossing the border into Canada at Sarnia, Ontario. My dad rolled down the window to speak to the border officer. He seemed surprised that anyone was out on the road given the conditions. We had not seen a car in a long time, so I imagine he hadn't seen a car for a while either. It was around 5 a.m. on Christmas Eve day. My dad handed over passports for him, me, and my sister. I had a pile of legal documents in my lap ready to answer questions. I assumed we would be pulled over and I would go through the paperwork inside. He looked at our passports and then said to my dad, "You gave me three passports but there are four people in the car." My dad told him the fourth person was his newest grandchild, my daughter. He asked my dad if he had a passport for her. My dad laughed and said that she was just twenty-four hours old and it was hard to obtain a passport at that age, because she couldn't sign her name yet. He looked at us and said, "Merry Christmas," and waved us through. That was it. I remember thinking that my dad would have made an amazing smuggler.

I had the most profound feeling of relief as we crossed into Canada. It felt like I truly exhaled for the first time in years. We had a few more hours ahead of us, but we were home.

Just after 9 a.m., we drove up the driveway to my parents' farmhouse. We brought Sadie inside to meet her family. My dad quietly went up to bed. I had never seen him look so tired. I could not have loved him more. He had not slept in over twenty-four hours. He had consumed many cans of Diet Coke over the eighteen-hour drive to stay alert. I did not know it at the time, but his socks and shoes were waterlogged after changing the tire. He had driven the last nine hours barefoot.

David and Georgia had to wait a few more hours to join us. The highway from Toronto was shut down because of weather conditions. When they arrived later that day, Sadie was napping naked on the enclosed front porch with sun shining down on her to help with her jaundice.

Sitting together in my parents' home with David, Georgia, Sadie, and my family, watching Mennonite carriages stream by on their way to Christmas Eve service, I was delirious with joy.

This was the moment that David and I had dreamed of.

It was here and it was spectacular.

CHAPTER TEN

"I Guess You Finally Relaxed"

WHEN DAVID AND I GOT MARRIED, I didn't care what I wore, what my hair looked like, or what kind of a ring I got. In fact, my entire wedding outfit cost less than the custom-made summer suit that David had made for himself. My sisters joked that the most expensive thing I purchased was my thong. My sister Sam did my make-up. When a friend weighed in on whether or not it looked okay, I remember her saying, right before she took over the job herself, "It looks great if you want her to look like a clown."

But our wedding vows mattered to me. If you were going to go to the trouble of making your relationship a marriage in the eyes of the law and inviting people to bear witness, then the promises you made to each other that day, in front of your community, were really important. We promised to stick with it for decades, through sickness and health, good times and bad times, joys and sorrows. I knew the dismal stats on marriage today and felt that we had odds as good as any other couple of navigating life to old age together. I remember making my way down my parents' walkway to join

David surrounded by our closest friends who stood with us. Our vows weren't just words. They were important commitments that we were making to each other. I felt like I understood their meaning. But in reality, I only came to understand what they meant in the face of the difficult events that followed, which tested those promises.

At the time, David was not working. A month before our wedding, he spent our honeymoon money (with my blessing) on travelling to Hawaii to play at the Ultimate Frisbee Club world championships. He was in the process of qualifying as a lawyer, which he had opted against doing when we graduated from law school a few years earlier, so he wasn't working. On paper he wasn't exactly the man my parents would have dreamt up for me. But as they watched us navigate the first few years of marriage, they came to love him dearly. They saw in David what I saw in him: his strength, his grit, his humanity, and his deep love and support for me.

He was, then and now, a talented athlete. I have always said that he lives life like he plays hockey. All substance and no flash. When the chips are down, he's the stay-at-home defenceman that you want on the ice.

Infertility, let alone losing a child, takes a toll on you as an individual. It also takes a heavy toll on you as a couple. David and I are both strong people who love each other, but that doesn't mean these experiences can't break you. Every relationship has a breaking point. There were a few times when I thought we may have reached ours. We were often white-knuckling our way forward. But our desire to always act in each other's best interests never wavered.

I used to joke that we were like the sitcom *The Addams Family*. The black cloud hovered over our doorstep and followed us wherever we went.

And then one day it was gone.

By that Christmas of 2008, we were raising two babies, born three months apart. We started to laugh again. We reclaimed friendships that had languished after Sam's death. We were rebuilding our lives and re-connecting with our community. But I was exhausted. David would come home from his work in a busy law firm and I would ask him to take over so I could lie down. I had started maternity leave when Georgia came home from the hospital and I had a nursing student at a nearby university helping out. Even with that help, I could hardly keep my eyes open during the day.

Shortly after Sam's death, a neighbour had left an anonymous note tacked to our fence admonishing us for the weeds in our garden. I almost wished I had a security camera to track down the person. But I had the last laugh. By the time we had the girls, our entire house was in a state of disrepair. Our windows were starting to rot so we had a painter come to strip and repaint them. He had a very thick Eastern European accent and I am a fast talker, so it was hard for us to understand each other. But through small gestures, like me making him a cup of tea or him helping me down the front stairs with my double stroller, we developed a rapport. He would look through the windows sometimes and see me sitting in my kitchen. I was usually contemplating how I was going to get myself up so that I could pick up the girls to change them, play with them, or feed them. He frequently asked me if I was ok. I realized that I must have seemed like a nice person but a terrible parent. Most days I could barely move.

At a certain point I knew I had to go see my doctor. I thought it could be mono. Maybe I was dying. Maybe I had narcolepsy. I knew, odds were, she would just say I was extremely tired because I had a three- and a six-month-old at home.

I scheduled a doctor's appointment.

I went to the pharmacy late one Friday afternoon to buy a pregnancy test. It seemed laughable but I knew that my doctor would ask the question before she ordered any tests. There was a time when I was such a "frequent flyer" with pregnancy tests that I wished I owned stock in companies that made them. In all those tries, dozens of them, I had never had even a hint of a pregnancy, not even the faintest line.

I felt almost embarrassed in the pharmacy that afternoon, as if people could see through me. I had not taken a pregnancy test in five years.

I went home. I took the test. And then I sat down on the edge of my bathtub and said out loud, "You have to be f--king kidding me." I was pregnant. It felt like the universe was messing with me. I waited until the following day, when my in-laws who were staying with us had left, to tell David. I wanted to be able to have a full conversation about this crazy news.

When David and I first started trying to have kids, I imagined different ways I would let him know that he was going to be a dad. They were all happy and playful. It seemed like such incredible news to be able to share with your partner.

In the end, six years after we talked on that balcony in Italy and decided to start our family, I sat him down for the most stilted and bizarre conversation we had ever had. I told him that I had taken a pregnancy test and that it was positive. I told him that we were having a baby. He thought I was joking. Once he realized I wasn't joking, he asked if I was sure that he was the father. He seemed genuinely confused. I confirmed that it was either him or the Almighty. Then we sat in silence for a long time in our kitchen processing the information.

I was at the end of the first trimester. We went to see my fertility specialist. We didn't know where else to go. We had always started at the fertility clinic, made embryos in a petri dish, transferred them to another woman's uterus, and then our surrogates would set up their own obstetrical care. We had never had a normal pregnancy experience. The doctor did a blood test and an ultrasound to confirm there an actual baby was in there. We learned that we were having a baby boy. Then he referred us to the obstetrician who had managed Debbie's pregnancy.

It still didn't feel real.

We kept the information to ourselves for a couple of weeks. I was working through in my head what the pregnancy meant for me personally and professionally. I was obviously happy but shocked. I was on maternity leave with the girls and planned to go back to work at the end of that summer, after ten months away. I would now be going back to work when I was five months pregnant. I wondered what my colleagues would say. I assumed people would question my ability to do my job. When I shared my concerns with my former boss, Karli, who by then was a close friend, she asked me if *I* felt like I could do my job. I said, "Of course." Then she gave me among the best advice I have ever received. She said, "Then go back and do your job. If someone has a problem with how you're doing it, they'll let you know." So that's what I did.

With surrogacy, there was no timeframe in which we needed to tell people about the pregnancy. But this time I was starting to show, partly because I had gained almost twenty pounds before discovering that I was pregnant. We sent the following email to our closest family and friends:

In the spirit of keeping things interesting, it appears that I am unexpectedly 12 weeks pregnant. Other than nausea, fatigue, and the onset of fatness things are progressing well. Have had a few ultrasounds and things look quite normal. If you're surprised, multiply that significantly and you'll approach what we're feeling. I am reasonably confident David is the father but have no recollection of events that might have led to this situation. On the upside, I am extremely confident I have not slept with anyone else. I may be carrying Jesus.

As I told David when I learned I was pregnant a few weeks

back, "If I told you I used to be a man you'd be less surprised than what I'm about to tell you." For those of you who thought I might actually be a man, it looks like I'll have the last laugh.

7 years, 4 surrogates, hundreds of thousands of dollars later and we'll end up raising 3 kids under the age of one. At least one of those kids won't have to find a talent we can exploit to pay off fertility bills. That child will be going to private school.

All is good. Will keep you posted and will likely chat with some of you in the coming days. Lots of love. Al

We got congratulatory notes from people. Friends who already had kids described all of the horrible things that would happen to my body, most of which involved some form of incontinence when I sneezed, laughed, or ran. The best emails we received were people congratulating us for still having sex with everything we had on the go at that time.

But most people, when they found out I was pregnant, said, "I guess you finally relaxed." If I had a dollar for every time someone said that, I would be writing this book on my yacht anchored off the Amalfi Coast. This line of thinking suggested that the problem all along was that I was just too uptight. I am uptight, but I don't think that was the issue. I'm no medical expert but scientific evidence also doesn't support the theory. Only a small percentage of women spontaneously get pregnant after adoption or unsuccessful infertility treatments. We just hear more about them when they do.

Mostly what I wanted to respond with was, "Have you lost your mind?' The least relaxing year we ever had was the year the girls were born. We navigated the arrival of a baby eleven weeks early, the disappearance, re-appearance, and eventual birth of another daughter in the United States, and then cared for two babies at home. David and I changed close to twenty diapers a day. We fed them every three hours around the clock and slept very little. I remember one night when they woke earlier than expected and I went downstairs to heat up bottles. I could hear David cajoling them in their bedroom trying to keep them calm. By the time I got upstairs they were screaming in his face like the exorcist. Just as we were about to put the bottles in their mouths one bottle dropped and rolled across the room. I tried to feed one, soothe the other who was hysterical by then, and watched David crawl around in the dark in his underwear trying to find the bottle. That was a pretty typical night in our house.

I have my own theory on why I ended up getting pregnant. David and I have known each other since I was twenty. Without getting into details that will make it even harder for my parents to read this book, let's just say that we've had many opportunities to make a baby over the years. I never got pregnant. But when we brought the girls home, beyond the huge emotional impact for both of us, my body had a very physical reaction to their presence in our house. My body ached. Not in a painful "I have picked up a baby thirty times today" way. More like a teenager going through puberty. Something hormonal was happening with my body.

Whatever it was, it created the conditions for me to get pregnant, once, and only once.

Fortunately, the world's most resilient embryo happened to come along just then.

CHAPTER ELEVEN

The Hat Trick

O F ALL OF THE THINGS that eluded me through infertility, I never felt that not being able to carry a child would leave a permanent wound. But I am grateful that, in the end, I was able to have the experience.

That said, I didn't enjoy pregnancy. None of my sisters did, which has always flummoxed our mother. She was basically pregnant from 1967 to 1975. She says she loved every pregnancy. If surrogacy had been possible back then, she would have been a great surrogate. She describes with flair the many activities she did during pregnancy, many of which would probably be outlawed today. She skied until the bitter end with my sisters Deb and Jen, who were February babies. She won a tennis match the night before I was born. She polished an entire brass staircase the day she went into labour with my sister Sharon. She fed half the neighbourhood spaghetti cooked over a fire in a blackout when she went into labour with my youngest sister Sam. She says she never felt stronger, happier, or more beautiful than when she was pregnant.

I did not have that experience. There was not a day during pregnancy that I enjoyed it. Between the nausea, gaining close to half my body weight, and the baby kicking my pubic area so repeatedly during the last couple months of pregnancy that I thought I would file assault charges, my body took a pounding. It was a daily grind. Part of me thought I should feel guilty for having those feelings, but I didn't. Given everything we had been through, I was just glad to be able to experience this like a normal person. Like me.

I may not have enjoyed it, but I felt fortunate to have a chance to experience it. I would never have relinquished this important role of carrying a baby to another woman unless I had to. It is a vulnerable feeling, leaving your baby in the care of someone else for an evening, let alone nine months. It is hard standing on the sidelines.

Because pregnancy happens every second of every day around the world, we treat it like it is ordinary, but I am so happy when I get an email sharing the news of a birth. So much needed to go right for that woman to get pregnant and for that baby to be safely delivered into the world. It is a triumph every single time. It is incredible what a woman's body can do.

In the weeks leading up to the birth, my due date couldn't come fast enough. I tried everything in my power to get the baby out earlier: sex, spicy food, Irish dancing, playing in a charity dodgeball game at work. Nothing worked.

The premier was hosting all of his senior staff for a pre-Christmas dinner at his house on my due date, December 20. I remember sitting as still as a statue on the very clean, very white couch in his living room, talking with his wife, willing my water not to break. I was mentally calculating how much money I would need to replace their couch. It turns out I didn't need to worry. The baby had battened down the hatches and wasn't going to be rushed out.

I saw my doctor on December 23 and he scheduled an induction for the next day. By then I was in physical agony.

Early the next morning, we drove to the hospital where they administered a drug to induce labour. Then they sent us home. My parents came that afternoon to take the girls to their farm for a few

days. We had just celebrated Sadie's first birthday. We fed her a cup-
cake in her highchair, the first time she had eaten refined sugar. She
took one bite and then looked up at us with eyes that said, "Where
the f--k have you been hiding this?" She was deliriously happy, which
made me happy because she and Georgia had no idea their world
was about to be flipped on its head.

If there is one thing that I have learned over the years with small
children, it is never to assume that any adult has eyes on them unless
they are specifically tasked with that responsibility. There is no such
thing as ten eyes are better than two eyes. A baby needs at least one
good eye on them at all times if they are mobile. We had all finished
a nice lunch. I had just walked back from the kitchen into the living room, where the girls had been playing surrounded by adults.
I scanned the room to locate Georgia, who was conspicuously absent.
There is a sound a baby makes when tumbling down the stairs that
sounds distinctly different from an object. You know it when you
hear it. I knew as soon as I heard the thump at the top of the stairs
that it was her tumbling down. She was at the bottom even before I
had a chance to reach the stairs. It was over in a few seconds. Other
than when she first came into the world screaming, I have never
been so happy to hear her cry. She was shaken but, fortunately, fine.
I thought of how much of life is just plain luck.

We packed up the girls. As we stood in our doorway hugging
them, I wanted to freeze the moment. This was the last day of our
first year together. It was exactly a year to the day that we had brought
Sadie home. It had been, without question, the best year of my life.

I walked for hours that day trying to bring on contractions.
Nothing happened.

We went out for dinner that night at a Japanese restaurant in our
old neighbourhood. The last time we had been there we had sat at
a table beside the actress Rachel McAdams, who was having a quiet
dinner with a friend. Throughout the evening, David repeatedly

dropped his napkin under her chair. She kept picking it up and giving it back to him, looking at me with an expression that said, "How are you with this guy?" I knew that she thought he was doing it on purpose. I knew that he had no idea who she was.

It was a bitterly cold night. It was also Christmas Eve so nothing was open. We bundled up and walked through the empty streets of Toronto. Most people were with their families. We walked a few kilometres to the hospital where Georgia had been in the NICU and dropped off chocolates for the nurses. It was the first time we had been back since we brought her home. We did not know the nurses on shift that night. We simply wanted to thank them for their work and for what they had done for our daughter. I looked at the different people sitting by their incubators. I knew how scared some of them must be. I hoped that their road ahead was as filled with joy as it had been for us.

We walked back towards the hospital where I would deliver and made a stop in an underground shopping pathway nearby to get out of the cold. Everything was closed but homeless people had moved in for the night. It was sad and sobering. Back outside we made our final trek to the hospital.

My water had still not broken but regular contractions had started.

I settled into a bed in the admitting area of the obstetrics wing and spent a lot of the night walking the hallways. David found a bed and slept. I could hear women asking the nurses if there was anything they could do to stop or slow down their labour so they could go home. Nobody wanted to be in there on Christmas. I didn't care when the baby was born, I just wanted him out safely.

I remembered that my sister Sharon had a very bad delivery with her twins and, at one point, had to take over decision-making from the medical resident, who was a doctor in training. I asked the doctor if she was a resident. She said that she was. I eyed her suspiciously.

She ended up being fantastic. She kept asking me if I needed an epidural. I kept telling her I didn't need one, but I made her promise that once I asked for one, she wouldn't leave me hanging. She finally asked why I was waiting so long. I explained that I didn't want it to wear off when I needed it most. She, in turn, explained that once the epidural was in, they could top it up for days. It wasn't time limited. I do not know where my understanding of how epidurals work came from but, again, it clearly wasn't from a medical book. She gave me one right away, which was good because it turned out to be a very long labour.

I told her that we had lost our first child in labour and delivery. I said that I didn't care how they got the baby out as long as he made it out safely. I told her that in sharing all of this she might think I was neurotic, but I needed her to know.

Thirty-six hours after they induced me, they finally wheeled me to the operating room for a C-section in the evening on Christmas Day. I was glad they had finally made that call. The baby and I were both fading. It was time to get him out.

But I started shivering uncontrollably. I thought I must be having a panic attack. My teeth were chattering so violently that I thought I might stop breathing. The doctors said that it was involuntary and sometimes happened in response to the drugs. They said it was perfectly normal and, yet, it felt like the least normal thing I had ever experienced. Then I blacked out. The next thing I remember was overhearing the nurses and doctors laugh about how big the baby was. Having just spent a day and a half trying to push him out of my vagina, his size felt like no laughing matter. He weighed, at birth, as much as Georgia and Sadie combined. He was ten pounds with a head the size of a basketball. We called him Lucas.

They cleaned him and swaddled him and then a nurse placed him in my arms. This was the fourth time I had held one of my babies. Every time was meaningful in its own way. This felt as close

to perfection as I could have imagined. David and I were experiencing this together, Lucas was healthy, the girls were safe with my
parents and we were in a regular hospital room five minutes from
our home.

The resident was going off shift when I was wheeled in for the
C-section. Before she left the hospital, she came to see us to make
sure the delivery had gone well. She had treated this birth like it
really mattered to her. I spoke with our obstetrician afterwards and
told him how exceptional she was. He said that she was the best
they had.

CHAPTER TWELVE

A New Normal

I N THE HOURS AFTER delivering Lucas, the nurses offered me Oxycodone to manage the pain. Even back then, Oxycodone had a bad rap. I learned later that the hospital dose is a much lower dose than the street drug. David and I don't drink alcohol or use drugs. I stopped drinking at eighteen. Going through university sober is not for the faint of heart, but I am glad I made the decision early enough for alcohol not to leave more of an imprint on my life than it had up to that point.

The night of Lucas's birth, David had convinced me that I might turn into a "lady of the night" if I took Oxy so when a nurse came by to offer me medication, I stoically asked for Tylenol. That was a mistake. She came back three hours later to check on my pain. She asked me on a scale of 1 to 10 how I was faring. I told her if a 10 was someone ripping my head off my body then I was at 9. I gratefully accepted the medication. I would have sold Lucas to her for some Oxy by then.

This time, unlike a surrogacy, my body had been through the wringer. All I wanted to do was sleep but Lucas wasn't going to let that happen. He was hungry and consuming food like a grown man at a hot-dog-eating competition. I had already made the decision to pump breastmilk and not breastfeed. I wanted Lucas to have breast-milk, but I definitely did not want to be the only feeder in the house. There was a woman floating around the hospital who kept trying to sign me up for the breastfeeding clinic. I told her I was all set with my plan. I had rented a breast pump from the hospital and I didn't need the clinic. She persisted. People have very strong feelings about breastfeeding. I am sure she worried that I wouldn't stick with it. I finally enlisted David to get her to go away. I had waited a long time to get to this place and I just wanted to be left alone.

I did cry for the first two weeks of pumping. Friends would tell me that it would get easier, which seemed hard to imagine. But they were right. One day the pain just stopped. After that, you could have shot a dart through my nipple and I wouldn't have felt it.

Lucas was doing well after the delivery, but I couldn't be dis-charged from the hospital until I had met certain milestones. Walking around was one. I tried to get out of bed the first day, but it felt like someone was tearing me in half. Peeing was another. I had had a catheter in for almost two days during labour and it was like I had since forgotten the mechanics of peeing. At some point, an extremely humourless nurse came by my room to tell me that if I didn't urinate in the next hour, she was going to put a catheter back in. Then she paused for emphasis and added, "without a seda-tive." That was enough to get me out of bed. I turned on faucets and mentally willed myself to pee, setting the stage for discharge.

We left the hospital on December 28 and my parents brought the girls back home.

It is hard to determine who was less enthusiastic about Lucas's arrival: his sisters or the neighbours. If he wasn't sleeping, he was eating, screaming, or pooping. Mostly screaming. We took him to the doctor who said that he had colic, which he would outgrow at some undetermined time. I couldn't pick up the girls that first week because of my C-section. They were clearly discombobulated. David was discombobulated. We all were. David had taken paternity leave, which I imagine he regretted immediately. The idea of our family was, at that point, infinitely better than the reality.

When the girls were born, David was the first man at his law firm to negotiate paid paternity leave. Eight weeks. As he was about to start, however, the decision landed on someone's desk who was apoplectic about its precedent-setting nature. The shit hit the fan and the decision was reversed. There was no way a group of men, many of whom had likely never changed a diaper, were going to sign off on a male lawyer being paid to be at home with his baby. I imagine they expected David would cancel his leave. He simply told them that, regardless of the money, the time with his family was non-negotiable. He was taking the leave.

Lucas' sisters and the neighbours had been unenthusiastic about his arrival, and now David's employer was unenthusiastic as well. David, again, was firm. We reflected on the fact that when Sam died, both of our workplaces had been immensely supportive. It was clear, then, that no one was going to pressure us back to work any earlier than we were ready—we could take as much paid time as we needed. It felt sad that the significance of one child's death was better understood than the significance of another's early life.

In those first few weeks, every time Lucas woke from a nap, we prepared ourselves for hours of screaming. If I could have found something other than a track suit that fit me, I probably would have hightailed it to work. But we hunkered down together, with our unflappable Irish caregiver, Suzanne, and managed three babies as best we could. It was the depth of winter and the girls caught a cold shortly after Lucas came home. I like to think they unintentionally gave it to Lucas, but we'll never really know without a polygraph. Once he became sick, he was clearly in distress and struggling to take a bottle. After a few days, I reluctantly took him to the doctor expecting to be told to wait out the cold. He checked Lucas and told me that he had bronchitis and may have pneumonia. I needed to get him to the hospital immediately.

I drove to the hospital in tears, with Lucas wheezing in the backseat. I brought him to the ER to have an X-ray done. His lungs were clear, which meant that he did not have pneumonia, but they put him on an oxygen level monitor and sent us home. We watched his oxygen levels closely day and night, and over the course of that week he got better. His size seemed to have inoculated him against potentially bad outcomes. At least one of us benefitted from the fact that he was born the size of a linebacker.

At his six-week check-up, our pediatrician suspected his colic was likely from acid reflux. We started him on baby antacids. He slept for twelve straight hours that night, only waking because I kept poking him to make sure he was alive. He has slept through the night ever since.

All my kids feel like a gift, but the main gift from my pregnancy with Lucas, other than Lucas himself, is knowing that I don't feel any differently about our children, regardless of whether or not I carried them. It may seem like a small detail, but I knew that I would spend the rest of my life answering questions from curious people about whether my bond with the girls was more fragile than my bond with Lucas because they were carried by another person.

Only through having a pregnancy could I know the answer to that question. I feel deeply connected to all of their births. Each was unique and memorable.

But my love for them is no different.

CHAPTER THIRTEEN

How Do You Put A Value On A Child?

M Y MOM WAS RAISED BY a divorced, single mother at a time when that was about as socially acceptable as being raised by someone running a meth lab out of their basement. She attended school in her small community with the children of her father's mistress. My dad grew up in a home with significantly more difficult circumstances than my mom, the least of which was very little money.

They didn't have easy childhoods, but they forged, together, a family life for me and my sisters rich with experiences and opportunities. It helped us grow into the people we became. They placed a heavy emphasis on values. You could eat a pack of Oreo cookies for breakfast in my house growing up and no one would blink. But you went to church on Sunday, you didn't swear (unless you were my mom), and you treated everyone, no matter who they were or where they came from, with respect. They built a great community of people around them, surrounding us with role models: kind, smart, loving, community-builders in their own right. They taught us to stand up for what we believed in and made us feel like our voices mattered in the world.

My mom used to say, "How on earth did we end up with five kids in seven years?" I imagine it began with a fairly tenuous relationship with birth control. But I am glad they did. My sisters and I have loved and supported each other through the many joys and challenges of our respective family-building experiences. Collectively we are blessed with fourteen beautiful children. We've had kids the old-fashioned way and through IVF, surrogacy, and adoption. We have kids with ADHD, Downs Syndrome, and Autism. We are a real-world example of women in our thirties having children in the twenty-first century. None of us had a linear path to parenthood. My sisters' family-building stories are theirs to tell but our shared destination led to this little posse of grandchildren.

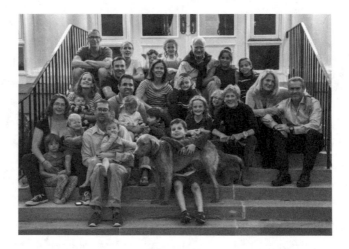

Our children didn't just change our individual lives, they changed our entire family.

Siblings can have pretty intense dynamics, but it is hard to describe the intensity of ours growing up. It didn't help that my dad would frequently bring home "presents" from his travels, like a pack of peanuts from the plane, and then absent-mindedly offer it to each of us. You would have thought it was a bag of gold bullion the way we fought over it. For all I know, my parents had us secretly enrolled in a behavioural studies research program.

With five girls close in age, someone was always nipping at your heels or hovering over you. None of us are quiet or laid back. We went to the same schools, did many of the same activities, and played the same sports. We bumped up against each other, a lot. We loved each other but we battled hard for space, for parental attention, and for our own independent identity in our family.

It was only when my older sister Deb started her own family, the first one of us to do so, that our relationships began to evolve.

Deb was in Columbia adopting her first child when David and I got married. A few weeks later, we gathered again at our parents' farm to meet her daughter, Emma. Holding her for the first time is an experience I will never forget. I was standing in the kitchen when Deb handed her to me, and she snuggled up on my shoulder and fell asleep. I felt such profound love for her and such happiness for my sister and for our family. My perspective shifted in that moment from looking backward at what our family had been to forward at what our family could be. Deb and I didn't have much of a relationship. We had carried many of our childhood grievances into our adult lives. But suddenly my mental ledger of the many ways in which I believed she had wronged me didn't seem quite as important. My main thought, as I held my niece, was that if I wanted a good relationship with her then I needed a good relationship with her mother. My sister and I went about building that relationship. Emma re-oriented our perspective towards the future. The impact of her arrival rippled across our whole family.

When my sister Sam called me early on in her second pregnancy to tell me that her child had the markers for Downs Syndrome, I did not know what to say. I followed her cues in terms of what she wanted from me as she worked through the information with her husband. A few weeks later, my sister Sharon and I took her away for a night at a spa. She was just through her first trimester and we knew she was tired physically and emotionally. We didn't know what head space she was in. She flew to Toronto from Boston, and we drove to a spa in the country and stayed up late talking and laughing in equal measures. She said to us that night that she had processed what she needed to process and now it was time to celebrate this child like we had celebrated every other child in our family.

Like Emma, Jane changed our family in subtle but important ways. She forced us to think about what truly matters. I had gone through something similar when we had Georgia. I wanted Jane to be able to build a happy life, grow into a kind and caring person, and contribute to making the world a better place. She is five years old and off to a pretty spectacular start.

I cannot imagine our family without Jane. I want to live in a world that appreciates what she brings into it.

We all grew watching our youngest sister embrace an unknown and teach us all so much about the power of inclusion.

That is the impact that children have.

I have always loved my sisters but having our kids made us better versions of ourselves. Even though we are spread across three different cities and two countries, we try to come together at least once a year at my parents' home for part of Christmas. We do this even though every year, without fail, someone's kid brings a terrible stomach flu. My children are a bit older now but when they were little and used to inflict every flu imaginable upon those around them, I often thought it was a miracle that any of us were still standing. My littlest nieces and nephews, my sisters Jen and Sam's kids, play that role now.

My dad held a unique position for a number of years as the Governor General of Canada. As part of the role, my parents moved into an official residence, a very large building that looked a bit like a small English palace. One of our first Christmases there, like clockwork, the stomach flu made the rounds on Christmas Eve. We also lost heat to the building that night. David spent most of it shivering, half-asleep, draped over the toilet bowl. No one was around to fix the heat so at some point, in desperation, one of us decided to light fires in some of the many fireplaces to try to generate warmth. Unfortunately, we forgot to open the flues, so we smoked out the building, setting off the fire alarms and bringing on a visit by the firefighters. Two years ago, someone tried to top that Christmas by bringing the stomach flu *and* head lice.

Still, there is no place in the world we would rather be than with each other.

I share all of this because it is impossible to begin to put a value on what children brought to our family. Or to quantify what children bring to individuals, communities, and countries in a way that captures their full impact.

I could have learned to live without a child. Infertility wasn't going to kill me. But it altered my life in profoundly negative ways.

And then *having* children altered my life in even more significant ways. The most surprising thing to me about having my children wasn't how much I loved them. It was realizing that that is how my parents must have felt about me. My dad used to say to me and my sisters several times a day, "Have I told you lately how much I love you?" We made fun of him relentlessly for this, but I do the same thing now with my kids. They respond exactly as I did at their age. Still, I can't help myself. It is just how I feel.

The love I have for them is more powerful than any feeling I have ever experienced. As a parent raising three young children, the oft-quoted phrase, "You are only as happy as your least happy child" resonates forcefully. Their hurts are your hurts, their fears are your fears. They are the centre of your world.

If I had to draw a link between how much we say we value children and the issue of infertility, I would say this: if having children is as precious, life-changing, and important as we say it is, then it is time we back that up through our actions and not just our words.

CHAPTER FOURTEEN

The Baby-Whisperer

I CALL MYSELF 'THE BABY-WHISPERER.'

I provide unsolicited family planning advice to women all the time. I am almost fifty now and when I hear a woman in her thirties talk about wanting to have a baby "one day," I tell her the facts. I tell her that her fertility peaked at twenty-eight and to go see her doctor to get a fertility work-up.

I do this with friends, with acquaintances, and with complete strangers. Occasionally I get a negative response: the baby-whisperer can come off as a bit bossy. But mostly women are grateful because few of them have heard any of this basic information before. Knowledge is power. When I run into some of these women later, we often have funny conversations. Usually they tell me they went home that evening and told their partner it was time to make a baby.

I wish someone had done this for me. If I had known the facts about infertility or the costs involved in getting help, David and I might have been more proactive about avoiding the path that we ended up on.

When women who are struggling with infertility reach out to me for advice, often referred through friends and acquaintances, I try to provide specific and practical information to help them hone in on the issues they need to consider. I have had so many of these conversations over the years that, early on, I developed a standard email that I send as follow up.

Here is what I tell them.

Get as much information as you can on your own fertility. Get your fertility work-up done.

A standard fertility work-up in Canada costs less than a couple of hundred dollars, is covered by public health insurance, and typically includes:

- A blood test to measure various hormones, including your Estrogen, Progesterone and Follicle Stimulating Hormone (FSH) levels. FSH is the hormone that tells your brain it is time to release an egg. The higher the measurement the harder your body is working to find a good egg, meaning your ovarian reserve may be low or your egg quality poor.
- An ovarian ultrasound to look at your ovaries and estimate how much you have left in there.
- A sono-hysterogram to look at the inside of your uterus and fallopian tubes to make sure there are no blockages or scarring that could impede pregnancy.

If you have a male partner, get him to do get his fertility work up done too. Have the results explained to you by your doctor so that you understand what they mean.

No one else cares as much about the outcome as you. Don't delay getting help. If you may need treatment then have your doctor refer you to a good specialist as soon as possible.

Understand the costs involved in treatment so that you know what is free and what help you can afford.

Time is not your friend. Don't keep trying the same thing over and over hoping this time is "the one". Know the facts and make decisions based on those. The clock is relentlessly ticking.

Most of my conversations about infertility are with women, but when it comes to surrogacy, all bets are off. The first time a man asked me to help him in his quest to have a baby, I burst into tears.

By that point, I had helped many women navigate infertility, but my friend Aaron needed the same kind of help. He walked into my office, sat down across from me, and asked me to help him and his partner Kevin find a surrogate . . . and I was overcome with emotion. I knew that the desire to be a parent, and the deeply painful experience of being unable to become one, was gender neutral. But I understood, in that moment, that surrogacy had opened up a world of possibility for many different people. I never expected my gay friends would be able to have a family. When I was growing up, most countries barred gay people from adopting. An option like gestational surrogacy (which has actually been around since 1985) was like something out of a sci-fi movie.

But surrogacy ended up being a "game changer" for me and for many of the people I have counseled—heterosexual couples, gay couples, and single people. I give them advice on how to find a good surrogate, information on doctors and fertility clinics that will work with a surrogate—because not everyone will—and details around the many costs and legal issues involved in Canadian and U.S. surrogacy. I often share my own surrogacy contracts (blacking out all of the identifying information for the surrogates) so that they can start to fully understand what is involved in this long and expensive process.

Through all of my conversations over the years, whether with women or men or anyone who asks for my help in trying to become a parent, there has been a single constant: I always tell them that whatever path you choose to try to have children, do everything you can to get to the end as fast as possible. The longer it takes, the harder it is. The greater the toll on every part of your life.

But if you are lucky enough to get to the end of that path with a child, I promise you it is magnificent.

CHAPTER FIFTEEN

My Truth

BELIEVE THAT SOME DEATHS ARE harder to accept than others. Some are almost expected. We prepare for them our whole lives. We know what to say and what to do when they happen. We are well-supported through grief and can make sense of them when they happen. But others are more confounding. They feel unjust. They change us as people, and it takes a long time to come to terms with the loss. Still others are almost unspeakable. There are no words of comfort or advice that help. They may break you. If you want to survive you just need to claw your way to the other side of your grief.

I have experienced these different kinds of losses through the deaths of three people in my life that I truly loved.

When I was twenty-five, my maternal grandmother died. She was a woman well ahead of her time. Faced with the choice of staying married to a serial philanderer or raising my mom and my aunt on her own, she made the difficult decision in 1948 to end the marriage. It took ten years and a private member's bill in parliament for her divorce to be legally recognized. In her mid-thirties, she went to university to get the kind of education that might lead to a job that could support her daughters. She became a social worker and spent much of her career working in remote communities in Northern

Ontario, flying around in bush planes. When she died, she had been retired for close to twenty years, but strangers wrote to our family or attended her funeral to share with us the impact she had on their lives.

She loved horror movies, so my sisters and I watched way more of those than we ever should have, or wanted to, when we stayed with her for part of each summer at her home in Sault Ste. Marie, Ontario. She made the best crustless grilled cheese sandwich and perfect breakfast sausage. She smoked a ton of Du Maurier Extra Light cigarettes. When she finally "quit" in her seventies, we would find her smoking in the bathroom. If one of us knocked on the door to confront her, with smoke literally pouring out from under the door, she would turn on the tap, spritz herself with air freshener, open the window and, when she emerged from the bathroom, look at you like she had no idea what you were talking about. She died at the age of seventy-nine, in a hospital room surrounded by the people she loved, saying the kind of goodbyes fitting for the extraordinary person that she was. As painful as her death felt, I also knew that I had been preparing for it my whole life. I knew that she was supposed to die before me. As much as anything, I just felt lucky to have been her granddaughter.

My second significant loss was my friend Timon. We met in high school. His family was a central part of the war resistance against the Nazis. After a failed coup against Hitler, they fled Germany, ending up in North America. Timon very much embodied his family's values, role-modeling in his life how to treat people well. He was like a brother to me. His wife, Mary, who I have known since we were children, is also one of my closest friends. They are Sadie's godparents and their daughter, Natasha, is my goddaughter.

At the age of thirty-six Timon was diagnosed with an aggressive and incurable form of cancer in his stomach. The four of us, me, David, Mary and Timon, carried each other through a lot over the next four difficult years. After he died, Mary asked me what it was like experiencing the loss as his friend. I told her that I missed him, which I still do. My heart broke for their two young children who would never have a chance to know their father the way they deserved to know him. His death felt unfair and unnatural because he was so young. But, as I described it, I knew that my grief must be so different from hers. I had a buffer for my grief: my own family. David and I had Georgia, Sadie and Lucas by then. The pain from the loss of my friend co-existed with the happiness in my own life and I could grieve from a secure place.

Losing Sam was very different. It destabilized every part of me. I had no buffer. David and I used to say that no matter how many people suffer with you, at the end of the day they go home to their own families, to their own lives. When it is your child, it is your life. There is no going somewhere else. At first, I didn't understand why it was so excruciatingly painful. I never actually knew Sam. But over time I understood that I was grieving everything that David and I would never have a chance to experience with her. Her death crushed us.

Navigating infertility with people—our families, friends and colleagues—had already been hard. Death took that to a whole new level. I knew how it must have felt for a lot of people trying to support us. They didn't know what to do. I felt the same way when Timon was diagnosed, almost paralyzed with fear, afraid of saying or doing the wrong thing. But I overcame my fear because the alternative. not being there for him, wasn't an option. I asked people who had experience with cancer for guidance. I tried to understand how I could help. As time went on, I grew more comfortable as a supporter.

Our friends and family felt truly lost about how to help us in our grief. David and I removed ourselves from much of our community over the course of dealing with infertility, largely to protect ourselves from interactions that drained us. After losing Sam, that protective instinct became a wall. We pared down our world to avoid anyone and anything that consumed energy that we desperately needed for ourselves. Everyone was doing their best, but most people didn't know what to say or do.

Conversely, what some people did and said, including funny, kind, loving, selfless things, I carry in my heart today. They marked me deeply as a person. I hope they helped me be a better supporter to other people going through difficult life experiences that I may not have had the experience to understand.

I am close with my family. What I remember most about experiencing this with them was the fact that they let me engage with them entirely on my terms. They made it all about me. I would disappear for weeks, sometimes months at a time. When I resurfaced, often only briefly to let them know that I was still standing, they were always there and would just let me know that they loved me. My sister Sharon sent me emails every few weeks with those exact words, "I love you," without ever expecting or receiving a response.

My family was always respectful of our privacy, but they also tried to understand what we were going through. My dad dropped by to see me at work one day and we sat in the building cafeteria having a tea. David and I had had a few failed IUIs and at least one failed IVF by then. I filled him in on where we were at with our infertility treatments. At one point in the conversation I mentioned that the doctor had introduced Viagra to my drug protocol. He didn't say anything but, as we continued the conversation, I thought, based on his follow up questions, that he may have assumed that I was taking Viagra to help with my libido. I explained that it was to increase blood flow to my uterus to build a better uterine lining for a baby to grow. I looked at him and said, "Between the two of us who would have thought I would be the first one on Viagra." We both laughed.

All of this was foreign to him not just because he was well into his sixties but because reproductive medicine and infertility had changed so much since my parents' generation had their kids. I knew a few kids growing up who were adopted. On the rare occasions where that kind of information was referenced in social circles it was spoken about in hushed tones, like it was a secret. Now one of their daughters and their son-in-law were making embryos in a petri dish and transferring them to another woman to carry. My parents were always open to learning, which helped them be there for us.

I witnessed something similar a few years later in another family. I was attending a caucus meeting where the proposed reforms around infertility and adoption that were being brought to cabinet for decision-making were being discussed. One of the caucus members, a retired teacher from a small Ontario town, got up to speak. Based on a lot of stereotyping, age, gender and geography, I assumed that he wouldn't understand infertility and expected him to be negative about the proposed reforms. I bristled even before he started speaking.

Then he started talking about how painful it had been to watch his daughter struggle with infertility. He spoke about his other daughter who offered her eggs to her sister. He couldn't believe this was possible and he was so grateful that it was. He talked about the grandchild that was born from this beautiful act. Then he endorsed the recommendations heading to cabinet. He didn't want other families to experience what his family had.

Beyond family, we experienced great love from friends, often in the unlikeliest of places.

Like my friend Bram who I had met practising law. When we were articling students, we used to walk home from the office each day debating which one of us our favourite law partner liked better (me). On the face of it, he was not an obvious candidate to be a caregiver to bereaved parents. He was a bachelor at the time, living a very social, single life. Our lives could not have been more different, but he bridged the gap between our two realities. He logged a lot of weekends in our kitchen, sometimes just sitting with us in silence. He figured out how to keep us company in a way that didn't feel intrusive but also made us feel less alone.

Today he is the godfather to our daughter Georgia. I got a call from him late one night a few years ago letting me know that their second child had died in utero at thirty-seven weeks. I was so shocked that my instinctive reflex was to think that he was joking. But the reality of his words sunk in quickly. I showed up at the hospital early the next morning and found him in the lobby with another friend. The three of us just cried.

David has a good friend named Mark who he met playing competitive Ultimate Frisbee. They represented Canada at the World Championships a number of times together. Mark is also an artist. For our wedding present, he gave us a beautiful painting of my parents' farm where we were married. Once we got caught up in infertility treatment and, eventually, grief, we lost contact with Mark. He lives in a different city so he would periodically reach out by phone or by email, but David was unresponsive. One day he appeared on our doorstep. He was in town and wanted to make sure we were okay. He said he half expected the blinds to be drawn and that David might turn him away. I had so much respect for him just showing up like that. The reality was that once we lost the thread, we didn't know how to find our way back to many people. It was a bit uncomfortable for all of us that afternoon, but his visit broke the ice and helped us find our way back into each other's lives.

I missed the chance to have my babies at the same time as my oldest and closest friends because it took so long to have mine. But I ended up having my babies around the same time as a beautiful group of work friends. This developed a second set of really close friends. Other than my three children, these friendships, to this day, are the great gift that came out of the journey. The common thread in this group, who gutted it out with me, was humour. They would start any conversation that involved them letting me know they were pregnant with, "I have terrible news." Then we would talk about how selfish they were. One day, having just left my office after telling me her news, I ended up in the bathroom alone with one of these women. When we realized it was just the two of us, she said, "Did you follow me into the bathroom to beat me up?" We both laughed. We owned the discomfort and labeled it for what it was.

Somehow laughter made things more bearable.

I remember walking in our house one evening a few months after Sam's death and hearing David laughing in the kitchen. It was such a welcome respite from grief, like finding water in the desert. I sat down beside him, in front of our television, and watched an episode of the show *Arrested Development*, for the first time, and understood why he was laughing so hard. We were basically unresponsive to all emotional overtures at that point but somehow humour broke through. I could have hugged the show's star, Jason Bateman. It is the closest I have come to writing a fan letter.

On the other side of infertility, it isn't the worst moments that I remember. It is the many acts of kindness that lifted us up. They had a deep impact on me. It is hard for me to imagine the kind of person who agrees to come to a hospital late one night, on short notice, and take photos of two strangers with their stillborn baby so that they will have a memory of her forever. Maybe he had his own experience with this kind of loss. I will be grateful for those pictures my whole life.

The funeral home where Sam was taken, embalmed and eventually cremated didn't charge for their services when it was for a baby. I was struck, even then, by the humanity of this gesture.

When the Scottish nurse tried to comfort me, I couldn't accept the overture in that moment. But I have often thought about what a gentle, compassionate and human act that was.

The list is long. My sisters offering to be our egg donors. Chella trying to be our surrogate. The ex-marine changing our tire. Diane's mom knitting Sadie's blanket. Debbie pumping breast milk for months after the birth.

I could not acknowledge many of these gestures at the time, which is sad, because I would have liked these people to know how much they mattered. Those acts of kindness are what has stayed with me. They helped me feel, in the darkest of times, that I was surrounded by love.

They carried me to the other side.

CHAPTER SIXTEEN

Closure

THE SUMMER I TURNED ELEVEN, I failed grade seven. Once I fell behind in French school, there was simply no way for me to catch up. I could hardly understand the teachers let alone the content they were trying to teach. When I got my final report card, no one, including me, was surprised. It had been clear throughout the year that I was not moving up to grade eight, barring an act of God. There was a well-known Cathedral near our house, the St. Joseph's Oratory. It had an imposing set of stairs, 283 to be exact, leading up a steep hill to the entrance to the building. Visitors often climbed the stairs on their knees in prayer. Near the end of grade seven, I went there one day. I climbed the stairs on my knees, in the pouring rain, praying that I would not fail. I didn't expect anything to come of it, but I didn't have much to lose.

There were many times throughout the years of infertility that I felt like I was back on those stairs. But the stakes felt so much higher. I would ask into the void, as if I was eleven-years-old again and still believed that someone out there was listening, "What can I do to get to the end of this?" "What do you want from me?" "What have I done?"

Somehow, when all was said and done, six-and-a-half years after we sat on a balcony in Italy, we ended up with three children in fifteen months. Our friends call them "The Triplets." Their births moved David and me beyond our grief over Sam and helped us rebuild our life.

Friends with young children would come to visit and joke that on their worst days they thought of me and would feel better. I would have three babies lying on the floor in an assembly line for diaper changes.

People would ask me if it was hard. My mom raised five girls. That was hard. One of my favourite childhood photos is taken in our kitchen in Montreal. Every cupboard is open. The counter is littered with the remnants of breakfast. Sharon, who is about eight, is on the floor making sandwiches for our lunchboxes, which she did every day. We called them "peanut butter and dog hair sandwiches" because we had a golden retriever dog who used to shed throughout the house and, on most days, you ended up with more than peanut butter in your sandwich. I remember one morning, we pushed my mom so far with our incessant fighting and messiness that she sat down on the floor in the middle of our front hall and started to spit out the banana she was eating. We called that The Day We Made Mom Spit Bananas. At the time, we wore the episode like a badge of honour. Now that we are all parents, she is having the last laugh. I have had my fair share of spitting bananas days.

I would simply tell people that it was busy. I knew "bad life" and I knew "good life." I would take the life I had, with three babies in diapers, any day of the week and twice on Sundays.

I made a conscious decision, once we had Georgia, Sadie, and Lucas, that I wanted to be happy, to fully and truly live the life that David and I have built. I couldn't let the fear of loss gain control over me.

Which, it turns out, is easier said than done. If you could experience for a day how much you were going to love your children before you had them, you might not actually have them. It is the most vulnerable feeling in the world. I don't know how much losing Sam impacted my experience of parenting. I have never felt that it made me a better or more loving parent. I think I am fundamentally the parent I would have been. I am warm, loving, and joke around a lot with my kids. I can also be impatient and, despite my children's best efforts to re-train me, I have what they describe as very "salty language," which they don't like. But losing Sam changed me as a person. It shaped my perspective on life well beyond parenting. I don't sweat the small or medium stuff. My main fears in life involve my children. But these can be intense. When it comes to the safety of the people I care about, I have always been prone to anxiety. My bedtime prayers growing up were exhausting. I worried that if I left someone out, they might be harmed.

I have often thought that losing Sam significantly magnified this underlying character trait. Once I had kids, I could have been persuaded that raising them in a bubble, in the countryside, surrounded by a twelve-foot fence was in their best interest. But my kids deserve the best mom I can be so I have to constantly balance my fears with the need to let them go so that they can grow into the curious, confident, and kind people I hope they will become. I have to remind myself when they're learning how to ride a bike to leave space for joy and not be consumed by what might happen if they veer into the street. Since the day they were born I kiss them every night in their sleep and say a silent thank you, to whoever or whatever might have a hand in all of this, that they made it through another day unharmed. That they are here.

On the face of it, my fears, I would imagine, are the same fears as many other parents. But the difference between fearing that something terrible might happen to your child and being able to recall the experience is big. That 'recall' is with you forever.

A few years ago, researchers studied a group of passengers who had been on a plane when it ran out of fuel mid-flight. The pilot successfully glided the plane to an emergency landing at a military air strip in the Azores but for an extended period of time, before the plane landed, the passengers likely assumed they were going to die.

In commenting on the research, a professor of psychiatry at Western University in Ontario said that "traumatic memories are not remembered, they're relived in a very vivid way. . . . In order to help a person heal from a traumatic event, the nature of their memories needs to be changed."

Having children after Sam changed the nature of my memories, and David's, too. Georgia, Sadie and Lucas allowed us to experience the beauty and fulfillment of being parents and not just sorrow. I don't think there is any such thing as closure when it comes to losing a child but with their births, we let go of the trauma of Sam's death and embraced a different, more hopeful journey.

We've never let go of Sam. I don't think of her every day or spend a lot of time wondering what she would have grown up to be. We will never know. But I wish more than anything in the world that she was here. Her memories are in a safe place. I can close my eyes and access them at any time. Sometimes I go back to the hospital room in my head. I hold out my arms and let the nurse place her in my arms so that I can hold her little body. I go there often—washing dishes, exercising, or just lying in bed—but I don't stay long. It is painful, and I don't want to live in pain. But I always want to be able to access that room.

My mom took Sam's ashes after they cremated her. I asked her to keep them safe until we felt that we could bring them home. I thought it would be a matter of months, but months turned in to years. Twelve years after she died, we finally brought her ashes home. I was alone in my parents' home, packing up from an end of summer visit. David and I had told our children about their own unique birth stories two summers earlier. But there was a significant part of our family story that we had not yet shared. I wanted to have something tangible in our house to connect them to their sister when we told them. My father-in-law, who is a talented wood-worker, made a beautiful small wooden box to hold Sam's ashes. It had sat empty on David's dresser for a number of years. Now it felt like the time to use it.

I had never seen Sam's ashes. I started to look around the house for something resembling an object you would keep ashes in. I guess I was looking for an urn. I assumed my mom would keep it in their bedroom. I rifled through drawers and closet shelves. At one point I feared that maybe the ashes had been lost. But then I looked across their bedroom and saw a small green velvet bag on my mom's dresser. It was tucked between a picture of my grandmother and my great-grandmother and a few of their belongings. I knew that velvet bag was Sam. I had expected something the size of a shoebox, but this was much smaller. I realized there wouldn't have been many ashes. There was a small white cardboard box in the bag with the following words written on the top:

Infant Sam Johnston Pickwoad
Cremated Wednesday September 6, 2006

I took the bag with me and placed it on the passenger seat of my car to drive back to Toronto with my other children in the back seat. I left a note for my mom in the place of the bag thanking her for keeping Sam all of these years and letting her know that we were finally bringing her home.

CHAPTER SEVENTEEN

The Other Side of Sorrow

M Y EXPERIENCE OF FAMILY-BUILDING is anchored in two competing truths. David and I would never have chosen the path we took to parenthood. It left battle scars and knowledge that we would rather not have. But that path also gave us Georgia, Sadie, and Lucas. It is impossible to imagine our life without them.

I don't try to reconcile these two unreconcilable realities.

I know I am one of the very lucky ones. I came out on the other side with a family.

Every night I get to tuck these three little Fruit Loops into bed.

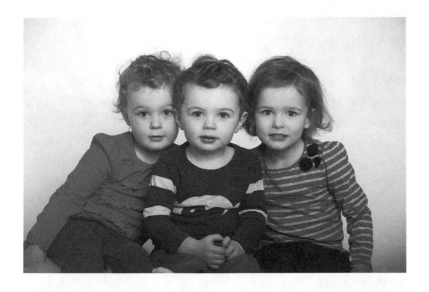

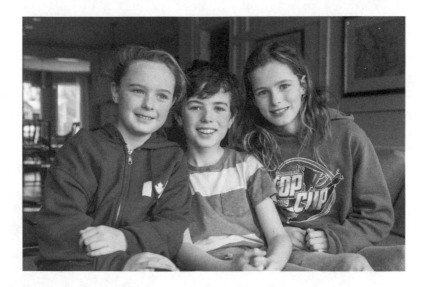

As our kids have grown it has become clear to me that I had har-bored two ridiculous assumptions before becoming a parent. First, that my kids wouldn't fight if I parented properly. It is almost embar-rassing to share that publicly.

My parents never (openly) judge our parenting but I am sure they chuckle as they watch us navigate their "not quite triplets but close enough in age to really cramp my style" sibling dynamics. My fam-ily seems genetically incapable of producing a laid-back offspring. I used to think my mom was joking when we would ask what she wanted for her birthday and she would say, "A day without fighting." Now I get it.

This connects to the second assumption, that our kids would be just like us. There are characteristics in each of them that I recognize in David and myself. But they are very much their own people. We have had to learn to parent them as the three very different individu-als that they are. Now that they are all in the double digits, I can really see the people they are becoming.

It is hard to remember that we once thought of Georgia as fragile. She was small enough to fit into the palm of David's hand when she was born but, at eleven, she is almost taller than me. I understand why she did so well in the NICU. They used to refer to her as a "smart baby." They weren't talking about her IQ but rather her abil-ity to pick up on and quickly learn the things that would help her grow. This quality still anchors everything she does. She is pretty fearless and open to new things. She plays on every sports team at school. She is a competitive swimmer. Last year she won the "spirit award" in her swim program for the best teammate and the "coach's award" for the most coachable athlete, recognizing two of her great characteristics—being a ferocious competitor and supporting others. She knocks my socks off every day.

Sadie is a totally different creature from Georgia. She does not like competition. She is very disciplined and puts in the time to become good at things on her own terms. She is a beautiful pianist and one of my favourite things is to watch her little fingers glide across the keys. When she is frustrated, or when things get loud and chaotic in our house, which they do regularly, she will often quietly slip away to play the piano. It seems like a form of catharsis for her. She is the peacemaker in our family and doesn't waste energy fighting. She's not a huge fan of change and despises unfairness. She is a deeply curious and caring person and when you look into her beautiful blue eyes, you can feel the strength of her character.

His sisters would give him, at best, a three-out-of-five-star rating, but Lucas is universally beloved. People at the kids' school sometimes stop me to ask if I am "Lucas's mom" and then proceed to tell me what a pleasure he is to teach or how glad they are that their child is friends with him. He has a confidence and joyfulness that I hope he never loses. He is a sporty little guy but an artist at heart. For his ninth birthday, the only thing more fantastic than watching him make and decorate his own cake was witnessing the elaborate unveiling for the fourteen nine-year-old boys in our kitchen. He assumed they would be as awestruck by the cake as he was. They just wanted to eat it. When I tuck him into bed at night, he makes me do a secret handshake, followed by a thumb wrestle, a round of "rock, paper, scissors" and capped off by a foot massage. When I turn out the lights and he tells me he loves me, I always say, "I love you so much more than you could ever love me." If he is a parent one day, he will understand.

At the end of the road that David and I took to have our children, we somehow ended up with these little characters.

I am grateful to David for so much, but especially three things. First, I never felt badly about my infertility. I used to joke that if David had known that I had ovaries like shrivelled prunes and the pregnancy potential of a menopausal nun, he wouldn't have given my dad as many goats. Part of how I felt about myself was how he made me feel. I always felt that he loved me and that we were in it together.

Second, when I decided to write about our experience building our family, he didn't bat an eye. If I was married to someone else and told them that I wanted to publicly air a lot of deeply personal information, including some of the most intimate details of our private life, I imagine some men would say, "Over my dead body. If you do that, I will leak every sex tape we ever made." Mom and Dad, that is a joke.

Finally, and most of all, he went the distance. I am not sure many men could have. But he never wavered. Going the distance brought Georgia, Sadie, and Lucas into our lives. They are the greatest happiness of my life.

I have included their birth announcements here.

It feels fitting to end with them.

Georgia Howell Johnston Pickwoad, September 22, 2008

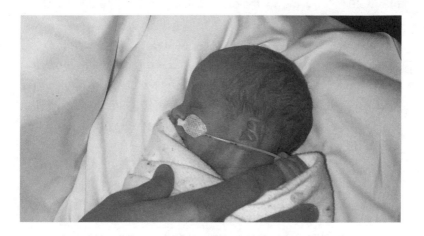

"As some of you may already know, on September 22, David and I became parents for a second time. Georgia Johnston Pickwoad was born at twenty-nine weeks, eleven weeks early, at Women's College Hospital. She came into the world just shy of three pounds, hollering like a banshee and is doing well in the NICU at WCH.

Georgia is still a wee thing but with each day looks less like a cross between a dried apricot and 10,000-year-old man and more like a small but healthy baby. She is described by the NICU staff as small and scrappy and they are delighted at how well she is doing for her age. She has been breathing on her own without assistance from the beginning, which is unexpected for twenty-nine weeks, and very comforting. She still has apnea where she forgets to breathe and sometimes needs a little tap on the back to remind her. She is on caffeine to stimulate her nervous system to help her with this. It's just a matter of time before she's demanding smoke breaks.

I attribute part of how well she's doing to the little toughie that she is but also to our carrier who took such good care of her for the first seven months, did everything she could to act in Georgia's best interests from day 1 and got herself to the hospital at the first sign of anything unusual to make sure that she and the baby were in good hands.

We look forward to bringing Georgia home likely sometime close to her Dec due date and daughter number three arriving sometime in December/early Jan. It has been a long few years getting here. We miss Sam every day and I don't imagine that will ever change. But two women have given us the gift of becoming parents again and that is the most precious thing we could ask for."

Sadie Johnston Pickwoad, December 22, 2008

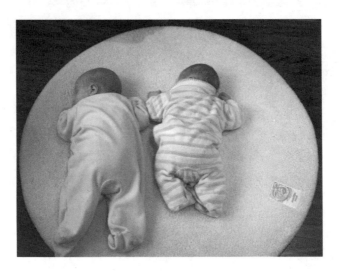

"On Monday December 22, Georgia's little sister, Sadie Johnston Pickwoad, was born in Green Bay, Wisconsin. Breaking with tradition, the delivery was uneventful. Fortunately, the weather was horrendous. Bringing home baby Jesus didn't hold a candle to this kid's homecoming. On day two of life Sadie embarked on a twenty hour road trip with her mother, grandfather, and youngest aunt through snow storms, sleet storms, rain storms, a twenty-five car pile-up on the highway, a flat tire in Michigan City, Indiana, just after midnight on the twenty-fourth and a 5:30 a.m. border crossing in Sarnia where the customs official is probably still wondering whether the infant in the back seat was kidnapped. All this and Sadie didn't even have the benefit of three wise men, a manger, or a barn full of hay to fall back on.

Notable highlights of the road trip included (i) me hopping into the back seat of the wrong SUV at a gas station in Chicago, mistaking a frightened older black woman for my father and (ii) my sister, Sam, trying to convince my dad to let Sadie drive because she was the most rested of us all.

2008 was a good year for this household. We look forward to so many things in 2009, not least of which is the chance to pawn myself off as a woman who recently had two children, never went up a jean size, and is overly solicitous with exercise tips for other women.

With much love to all of you for the New Year."

Lucas Christopher Johnston Pickwoad, December 25, 2009

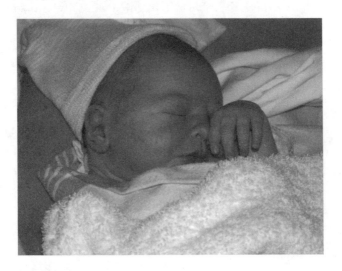

"I wanted to let you know that David and I welcomed baby Lucas (Lucas Christopher Johnston Pickwoad) into the world on December 25th. He is a healthy and huge ten-pound boy. After twenty hours of labour and a C-section, he's lucky his name isn't "attempted man-slaughter." There has been wide speculation this kid may be baby Jesus. On first blush, it seems unlikely, but there is some compelling evidence:

- Four words: immaculate conception miracle child. David is still contemplating a paternity test.
- I may not be the strongest contender to succeed Mary but I could plausibly crack the top 100 list. I went to church growing up. After a summer of partying in France my parents sent me to bible camp.
- Have I mentioned Lucas was born on Christmas . . . with a peach fuzzy beard and wearing a loin cloth.
- He speaks Latin.

Only time will tell. But we plan on treating him better than his sisters, just to be on the safe side. Wishing you a great holiday and wonderful 2010."

EPILOGUE

Policy is Personal

FOR MANY YEARS, my dad routinely summarized, in broad strokes, the church sermon on Sunday and emailed it, in real time, to me and my sisters. Usually we would tell him to put down his device in church. His fellow parishioners must have thought he was playing Angry Birds. One Sunday, he sent us a summary of a sermon on the theme of serving others. He included personal reflections about how proud he was that we had all gravitated to work that was in the service of others. My sister Sam responded, "True, but the same could be said if we were hookers."

The only thing my sisters and I enjoy more than laughing at our own jokes is a vigorous policy debate. We have all built our professional lives around some form of public policy work.

I have focused my advice in this book on women and the simple, actionable things they can do, because women are their own (and often only) best line of defence when it comes to protecting their choices around parenthood. I speak often and passionately about infertility because it is an important health issue for women to be aware of.

But for real change to happen we need much more than individual action. We need powerful agents—governments, businesses and doctors—to become fully engaged with this issue for broad and impactful policy change.

If I learned anything in my job in government, it is that bringing about policy change, around any issue, is really hard. Decision-makers need to care enough to take up the mantle in the first place.

Policy making is a deeply personal process. People who make and shape policy are real people, wrestling with real issues. Beyond the research and facts underpinning policy development, it is decision-makers' emotions, experiences, values, and biases that create policy. When it comes to what issues get championed behind closed doors, these issues are typically relevant to the people behind those doors.

I experienced this up close and personal when I was advocating for changes to infertility policy. In the lead-up to the 2007 election, I was asked to develop policy proposals that supported women for our election platform. I saw an opportunity to get infertility on our policy agenda. Most of the decision-makers in these discussions were men in their forties and fifties for whom the issue of infertility had little personal appeal. But a small group of us in our thirties, who had direct experience, advocated for it. After much back and forth over many weeks, something relatively small—a commitment to set up a panel to look at the issue of infertility—was included in the platform. As small as it was, it felt like a victory, as it would bring this issue out in the open during an election campaign.

However, shortly before the platform was put to bed, a colleague let me know that the premier no longer wanted to include it. I thought my head might pop off. I was furious. I felt that the biases of older men were derailing an opportunity to do something important for women, especially younger women. To make matters worse, I could tell that people thought I was so angry because of my own personal experience. As if this was about me.

One of the great qualities of the premier was that he was open to different perspectives and hearing people out. I believed in this policy proposal so I tried to understand his objections so that I could address them. His main objection came down to one question: "If this is such a big deal for women, why am I not hearing about it?" He had consulted his mother in her eighties, his wife in her fifties and his daughter in her twenties, and this issue was not very relevant to them.

But I knew they were the wrong age groups to understand the issue. I told him that stereotypes around infertile women, blame and shame, and old science, including very outdated success rates for treatment, were holding back the discussions that we needed to have. I said that infertility was all around him in our office, which surprised him.

I had travelled with him for a week earlier that year while I was in the middle of an IVF cycle. I brought a doctor's note in case I needed to explain my IVF medication going through airport security. Somehow, I still can't bring a nail file on a plane but that week a dozen needles and vials full of injectable hormones didn't raise any alarm bells. I had to discreetly inject myself on airplanes and in airport, hotel, and restaurant bathrooms all week long. It would never have crossed my mind to share what I was going through with the premier. I wasn't uncomfortable talking about my infertility, I just didn't think he needed to know that I was trying to have a baby.

Some women in our office who also had first-hand experience with infertility went to speak with him directly to share their stories. To his credit, he was persuaded and signed off on including something in the platform:

> Help people have families by making fertility monitoring available earlier in life, so people know whether or not they are likely to have a problem having children and make treatment and adoption more accessible and affordable for people.

Soon after the election victory, the government convened an expert panel of Ontarians to make recommendations around the platform commitment. The day the panel was announced, I went home in the evening, got into the shower, and cried. It felt like we might actually get somewhere on the issue.

The chair of the panel was a sixty-six-year-old man, a well-respected university president at the time, with a background in securities law. Some people were perplexed by his decision to take this issue on. He accepted for two reasons. First, because he was my father, and I asked him. Barring wildly inappropriate requests, he is predisposed to say yes to his kids. In retrospect, I probably should have pushed the envelope further than I did growing up.

Second, he had enough of an understanding of the issues; he watched my sister Deb go through the adoption process and me struggle through infertility treatments. He knew how important it was to get this right. The issue was personal for him and for many others on the panel.

The report the panel delivered to government twelve months later, *Raising Expectations*, is one of the most thoughtful and compelling reports I read on any issue while I was in government. The overarching ambition was to make Ontario the best place in the world to build a family.

I think every country should have that ambition.

The panel advocated for more public funding for infertility treatment, including funding for awareness raising, fertility monitoring, and IVF. It advocated for better support for people pursuing international and domestic adoption, including significant changes to make it easier for children in foster care to find permanent homes.

The report made the case not just around fairness and values, which is where you might have expected the panel to go. Instead, it drew a clear link between the proposed changes and the specific benefits, including significant cost savings and improved outcomes for parents and children that would come through better public policy around adoption and infertility treatment.

The recommendations were supported by a thorough and compelling economic and cost-benefit analysis. The changes would be cost neutral or generate savings for the public health system. This was important because framing this as an economic issue, even more than a moral one, was to me the only way the proposed recommendations could get traction in government. Governments have finite resources and many competing demands for those resources. Helping people see that something is not just "the right thing to do" but also the economically "smart thing to do" is hugely helpful to move a policy forward.

The report did that. It showed that it cost $32,000 a year to keep a foster child in care but significantly less to provide supports and subsidies to help families give children permanent homes. It made clear that multiple births, twin and triplet pregnancies, are seventeen times more likely to be pre-term, to require a caesarian delivery, and to need expensive care at birth and throughout their lives, placing a significant cost burden on public health care. At the time of the report, babies born from assisted reproduction made up 1% to 2% of all live births in Ontario but, because of the high rate of multiple births, accounted for 20% of all babies admitted to the NICU each year. The report hammered home the points, through evidence and analysis, that it costs more to care for multiples than to prevent them. It estimated that, by funding IVF, "Ontario could save the health system $400-$550 million over the next ten years by reducing the number of multiple births born from assisted reproduction and another $300-$460 million in savings that would have been spent on extra support for these children over their lifetime." Investing in IVF would reduce the rate of multiple births by reducing the reliance on inexpensive options like IUI and Clomid, which stimulates the production of many eggs, and also reduce the practice of transferring multiple embryos with IVF hoping that at least one will take.

The report established that the single greatest barrier preventing lower- and middle-income people from accessing the safest and best options to build their families was money.

It helped Ontarians understand that the existing approach was about cleaning up problems rather than preventing them in the first place. The recommendations, to me, were a no brainer.

But one can never underestimate resistance to change.

Obstacles in moving the policy work forward came primarily from one senior health bureaucrat, a fifty-something male who was one of the key gatekeepers in the policy-making process. He did not see infertility as an important policy issue. He worked hard to undermine the report recommendations, to cloud the issues and put a smokescreen around the empirical cost benefit evidence. This made it harder to get the clarity, consensus, and conviction necessary to drive change.

When the report recommendations came to the provincial cabinet a couple of years later, in 2010, there was little appetite to do more around infertility among ministers, unsurprisingly. They didn't seem opposed so much as indifferent. Most were in their fifties and sixties and had little personal experience with or understanding of the problem.

But the infertility discussion continued inside government well after I had left. In April 2014, the government announced that Ontario would begin funding one cycle of IVF for women under the age of forty-three, including women acting as surrogates. As the expert panel had predicted, the Canadian rate of multiples has plummeted from a high of over 30% of IVF births in 2009 to under 10% by 2017, in part because of Ontario's policy change.

Most importantly, the policy was inclusive. It reflected an important evolution in how we define "family," recognizing that single people and same sex couples should have the same access to help to build their families as a heterosexual couple like David and me. It reflected the world we live in today.

By the time the policy change was announced, it had taken seven years and many hands. The facts and data had not changed during the intervening few years since the initial cabinet discussion. But the context in which the discussions were happening changed. By 2014, there was a much deeper personal connection to the issue inside government. Two of the main proponents were men in influential, senior roles working for the premier who had needed infertility treatments to have their families. They championed this issue behind closed doors.

As well, the cabinet demographics had evolved, with more women and younger people around the table. There was a female minister of health shepherding the policy through government. There was a female premier, also the first openly-gay premier in Canada.

Different perspectives were shaping the policy development and decision-making than what had been the case a few years earlier. The policy had become more personal.

I share this particular anecdote to illustrate that even with compelling facts, evidence and advocacy, it still took a small village for this change to happen.

* * *

The stakes for women are too high to simply allow the issue of infertility to be ignored. The majority of babies in many countries are now born to women in their thirties, so we need to adapt to the realities that go along with that. Our public and health policy related to infertility needs to evolve.

Governments have a crucial role to play. More than half of the countries in the world now have fertility rates below the population replacement level; despite these plummeting fertility rates, most countries offer little or no public funding for fertility treatments like IVF.

I find it hard to reconcile the excitement that people feel about children with how completely disinterested we seem to be in helping people have children. If governments truly value children the way many say they do, then family-building policies should be high up on their public policy agenda.

Yet, in Canada, only five of ten provincial governments offer any public funding at all. As a potential sign of progress, however, Quebec just re-instated funding for IVF after cancelling its program in 2015 and, starting in January 2021, PEI is funding IVF for the first time. Only a handful of state governments in the United States mandate IVF coverage as part of insurer benefits.

However, governments in countries like Australia, France, Belgium, Italy, Spain, Israel, the Netherlands, Norway, and Sweden have offered substantial public funding for IVF for many years. Their experiences investing public money in IVF are examples that we can learn from.

* * *

Businesses also have an important role. They provide health benefits to millions of employees around the world. Including coverage for a specific drug, health service, or treatment in a health plan can literally change lives. Including fertility benefits in these plans can be the difference between having a child and not.

In 2014, Facebook and Apple were the first companies in the world to offer health benefit coverage for egg freezing and, in Apple's case, for surrogacy as well. These companies were outliers at the time. But in January 2019, the *New York Times* published an article, "I.V.F. Coverage Is the Benefit Everyone Wants", sharing data showing an increase in the number of companies offering fertility benefits and an increase in the amount of those benefits. Procter and Gamble Company, for example, moved from $5,000 in fertility benefits in 2017 to $40,000 in 2018.

This speaks to progress but the truth is that the majority of women don't work in Fortune 500 companies, so access to the kinds of health plans that might include fertility benefits is very narrow.

* * *

Finally, doctors have an essential role to play. Women are still surrounded by misinformation. The Public Health Agency of Canada, overseen by Canada's Minister of Health, advises on its website that women should try conceiving for twelve months before seeking help if they are under thirty-five. Given the actual facts around fertility I can't understand how anyone would offer that advice to women today.

Doctors should make fertility counselling and monitoring routinely available to women as part of their annual check-up.

Tracking my fertility as part of my annual medical check-up would have flagged that my fertility was declining much faster than the "average" woman. It would have given me important facts about my own body to help me make informed decisions, like whether to freeze my eggs or start trying earlier. I doubt that David and I would have started much earlier but we could have avoided a futile and painful year of trying to conceive on our own if we had known that my fertility was already compromised. Losing precious time before seeking help made our path to parenthood that much harder.

I know that this can be a hard conversation to have with a woman. I can imagine doctors getting a less than receptive response if they raise the issue proactively with some patients. But a more perilous scenario is one where a woman loses her choice.

Talking about fertility can be a life-altering conversation and doctors are uniquely positioned to have it.

DEDICATION

PEOPLE HAVE ASKED ME if writing about my experience with infertility was a form of catharsis. It wasn't. I worked through what I needed to long ago. Telling my story is about advocacy.

I have shared my journey openly and honestly, the sadness and sorrows, the full financial and emotional costs, the joys and triumphs, the good and the bad, hoping that no single anecdote or piece of information overshadows the main message in this book, which is that change is desperately needed. Not for me or women my age. Our window has closed. It's for women who have yet to build their own families. They deserve much more than our stories. They need concrete actions.

I have the story that I do for many reasons, including strength and perseverance, incredible advances in reproductive medicine and technology, the skill and care of two great fertility specialists, Dr. Fay Weisberg and Dr. Cliff Librach, and the great fortune to have been able to afford help. But, as much as anything, I have the story that I do because of Diane and Debbie. They came into our lives and found two very broken people. They chose to embark on this journey with us. I do not know how my story would have turned out if it weren't for them. I am glad I never had to find out.

It is hard to find words to express the love and gratitude you feel for a woman who carries your child. Diane and Debbie live in a unique place in our hearts.

This book is dedicated to them.

ACKNOWLEDGEMENTS

I N THE FALL OF 2018 I decided that I wanted to write a book about infertility.

I have done a lot of writing throughout my professional life but I had never written a book so I asked two friends, Gill Deacon and Amy Stewart, who have both written multiple books, for advice. They said, "you need to speak to Sam Haywood". Sam is the head of Transatlantic Agency and also their book agent. Sam kindly agreed to meet me for coffee one morning to give me advice. Even better, she emailed me that night to say that she would take me on as a client. This book would not have been possible without Sam's encouragement, editorial guidance and honest feedback.

Once I had a good first draft manuscript my friend Sara Angel connected me to Dianna Symonds, the former editor of Saturday Night Magazine, to ask if she would consider editing my manuscript. Dianna and I did not know each other personally but she became an invaluable editor and writing advisor. She chopped, finessed and re-arranged sections and made the manuscript so much better. She would not accept payment for her incredible work. I am grateful to her for that but even more for helping me become a better writer.

I was very lucky for the continuous input and encouragement of my dad and my husband from beginning to end. An enormous thank-you as well to Karli Farrow, Susannah and Haining Gouinlock, Deborah Gillis, Mary Gallery, Elizabeth McInnes, Chella Tingley and Georgia Drummond for providing invaluable feedback on the manuscript and, a very special thanks to Bill Downe, who may not have put this book topic on his Christmas list but provided comments that were as insightful and thoughtful as any I received throughout the process.

I want to acknowledge Ken Whyte. The difference between a manuscript sitting in a closet collecting dust and seeing the light of day is a publisher. You are a fantastic writer and editor. I feel very fortunate to have been able to do this book with you and with Sutherland House.

My final thanks are to Georgia, Sadie and Lucas, my three great loves and the most important part of my story, of my life.

I don't know how you will remember your mother when you grow up but watching me work will be one memory—hopefully it won't be the defining one. When you are old enough to read this book, I hope you will feel like I have done justice to your birth stories.

NOTES

1 "Fertility: Fewer children, older moms," *Statistics Canada*, May 2018.

2 "Canada's total fertility rate hits a record low," *Statistics Canada*, September 2020.

3 Claudine Provencher, et al., "Fertility: Overview, 2012 to 2016," *Statistics Canada*, June 2018.

4 Joyce A. Martin, et al., "Births: Final Data for 2016," *National Vital Statistics Reports*, 67.1, January 2018.

5 Gretchen Livingston, "For most highly educated women, motherhood doesn't start until the 30s," *Pew Research Center*, January 15, 2015.

6 Annual Report from Canadian Fertility & Andrology Society (CFAS), 2001 based on the Canadian Assisted Reproductive Technologies Register (CARTR).

7 Annual Report from CAFS, 2017 based on the CARTR.

8 Data taken from the Canadian Centre for Disease Control & Prevention 2017 Fertility Clinic Success Rates Report.

9 Information taken from private market analysis companies, including "In-Vitro Fertilization Market Size, Share & Trends Analysis Report By Instrument (Disposable Devices, Culture Media, Capital Equipment), By Procedure Type, By End Use, By Region, And Segment Forecasts, 2020-2027," *Grand View Research*, February 2020.

10 "Age of mothers at childbirth and age-specific fertility," *OECD Social Policy Division*, SF2.3, May 2019.

11 "Female Age-Related Fertility Decline," *The American College of Obstetricians and Gynecologists Committee on Gynecologic Practice*, 589, March 2014.